CARLYLE JANSEN

W0082009

SEX YOURSELF

"We women have had our minds filled with negative messages, especially about female pleasure. It's time to own our sexuality and this book helps you do it! Carlyle covers all the bases—no female body part nor question has gone unturned or unanswered. I loved every page and it will be on my must-read list for clients."

—Laurie Betito, Ph.D., author of *The Sex Bible for People Over 50*

THE **WOMAN'S GUIDE** TO **MASTERING MASTURBATION** AND **ACHIEVING POWERFUL ORGASMS**

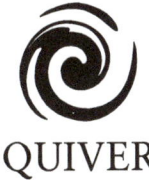

QUIVER

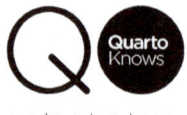

Brimming with creative inspiration, how-to projects, and useful information to enrich your everyday life, Quarto Knows is a favorite destination for those pursuing their interests and passions. Visit our site and dig deeper with our books into your area of interest: Quarto Creates, Quarto Cooks, Quarto Homes, Quarto Lives, Quarto Drives, Quarto Explores, Quarto Gifts, or Quarto Kids.

© 2015 Quiver
Text © 2015 Quiver
Illustrations © 2015 Quiver

First published in 2015 by
Quiver, an imprint of
The Quarto Group,
100 Cummings Center,
Suite 265-D,
Beverly, MA 01915, USA.
T (978) 282-9590 F (978) 283-2742
www.QuartoKnows.com

The Publisher maintains the records relating to images in this book required by 18 USC 2257. Records are located at Quarto Publishing Group USA, Inc., 100 Cummings Center, Suite 265-D, Beverly, MA 01915-6101.

All rights reserved. No part of this book may be reproduced in any form without written permission of the copyright owners. All images in this book have been reproduced with the knowledge and prior consent of the artists concerned, and no responsibility is accepted by producer, publisher, or printer for any infringement of copyright or otherwise, arising from the contents of this publication. Every effort has been made to ensure that credits accurately comply with information supplied. We apologize for any inaccuracies that may have occurred and will resolve inaccurate or missing information in a subsequent reprinting of the book.

Quiver titles are also available at discount for retail, wholesale, promotional, and bulk purchase. For details, contact the Special Sales Manager by email at specialsales@quarto.com or by mail at The Quarto Group, Attn: Special Sales Manager, 100 Cummings Center, Suite 265-D, Beverly, MA 01915, USA.

ISBN: 978-1-59233-679-1

Digital edition published in 2015
eISBN: 978-1-62788-354-2

Library of Congress Cataloging-in-Publication Data

Jansen, Carlyle.
Sex yourself : the woman's guide to mastering masturbation and achieving powerful orgasms / Carlyle Jansen.
pages cm
ISBN 978-1-59233-679-1 (paperback) –
ISBN 978-1-62788-354-2 (eISBN)
1. Sex instruction. 2. Sex. I. Title.
HQ56.J275 2015
613.9071--dc23
2014049443

Cover design: Burge Agency
Book design: Burge Agency
Illustrations: Laia Albaladejo
Photography: Shutterstock.com
Developmental edit: Megan Buckley

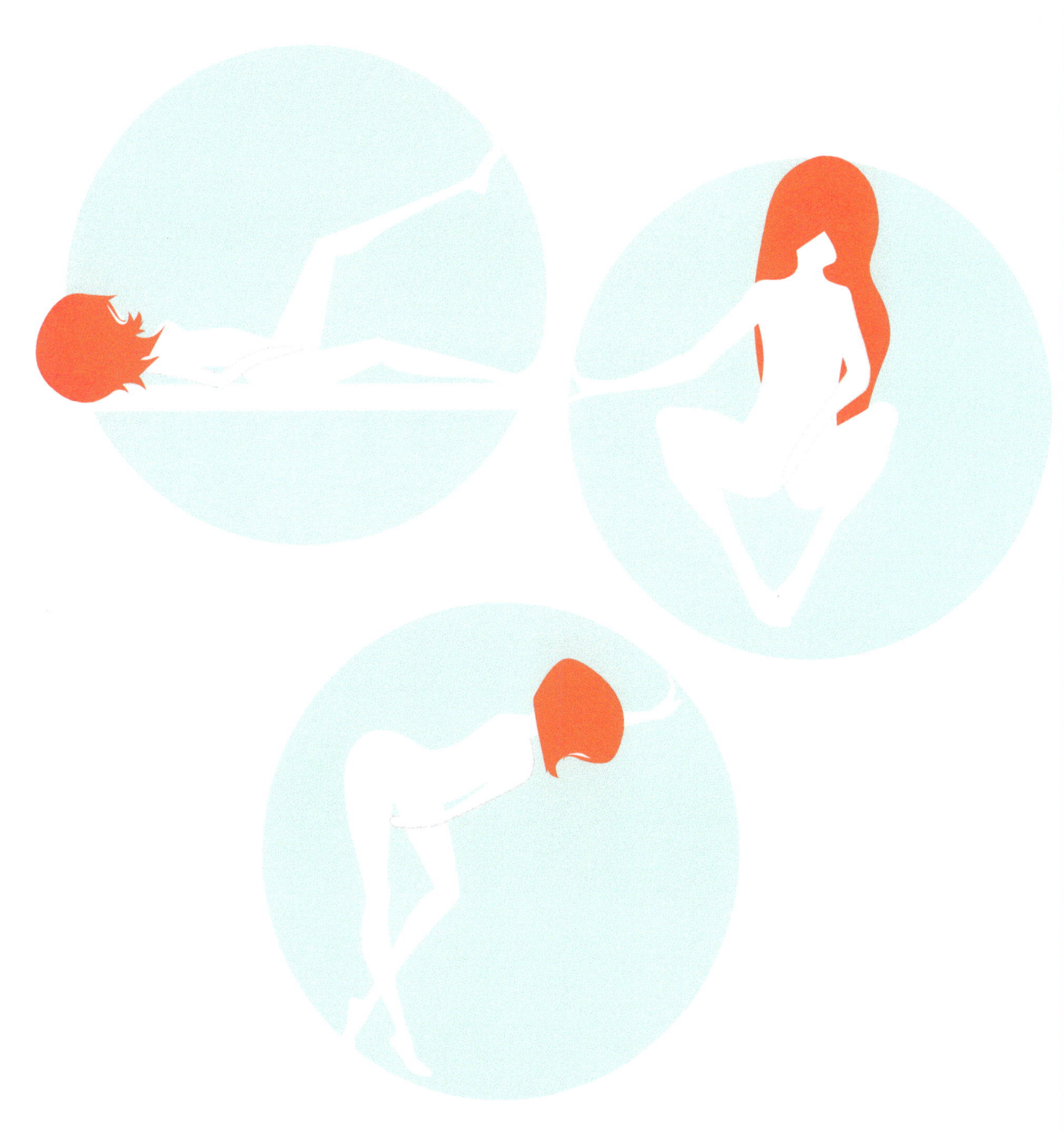

CONTENTS

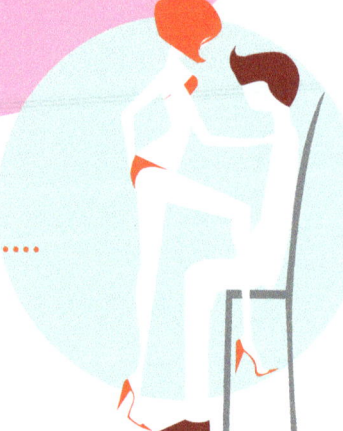

INTRODUCTION   6

CHAPTER ONE
HEALTHY SOLO SEX   12

CHAPTER TWO
ANATOMY, HOT SPOTS, AND EROGENOUS ZONES   22

CHAPTER THREE
KICK-STARTING PLEASURE:
DISCOVERING YOUR EROTIC POTENTIAL   42

CHAPTER FOUR
HOW TO SHE-BOP:
STROKES, TECHNIQUES, AND TRICKS   62

CHAPTER FIVE
CHOOSING AND USING SEX TOYS   88

CHAPTER SIX
SPICING IT UP:
KEEP YOUR SOLO SEX ROUTINE FUN, HOT, AND EXCITING   112

CHAPTER SEVEN
BIGGER, BETTER, MULTIPLE ORGASMS   124

CHAPTER EIGHT
COMING TOGETHER:
FROM ORGASMS ALONE TO ORGASMS WITH A PARTNER 150

CONCLUSION   166

RESOURCES   168

REFERENCES   170

ABOUT THE AUTHOR   172

ACKNOWLEDGMENTS   173

INDEX   174

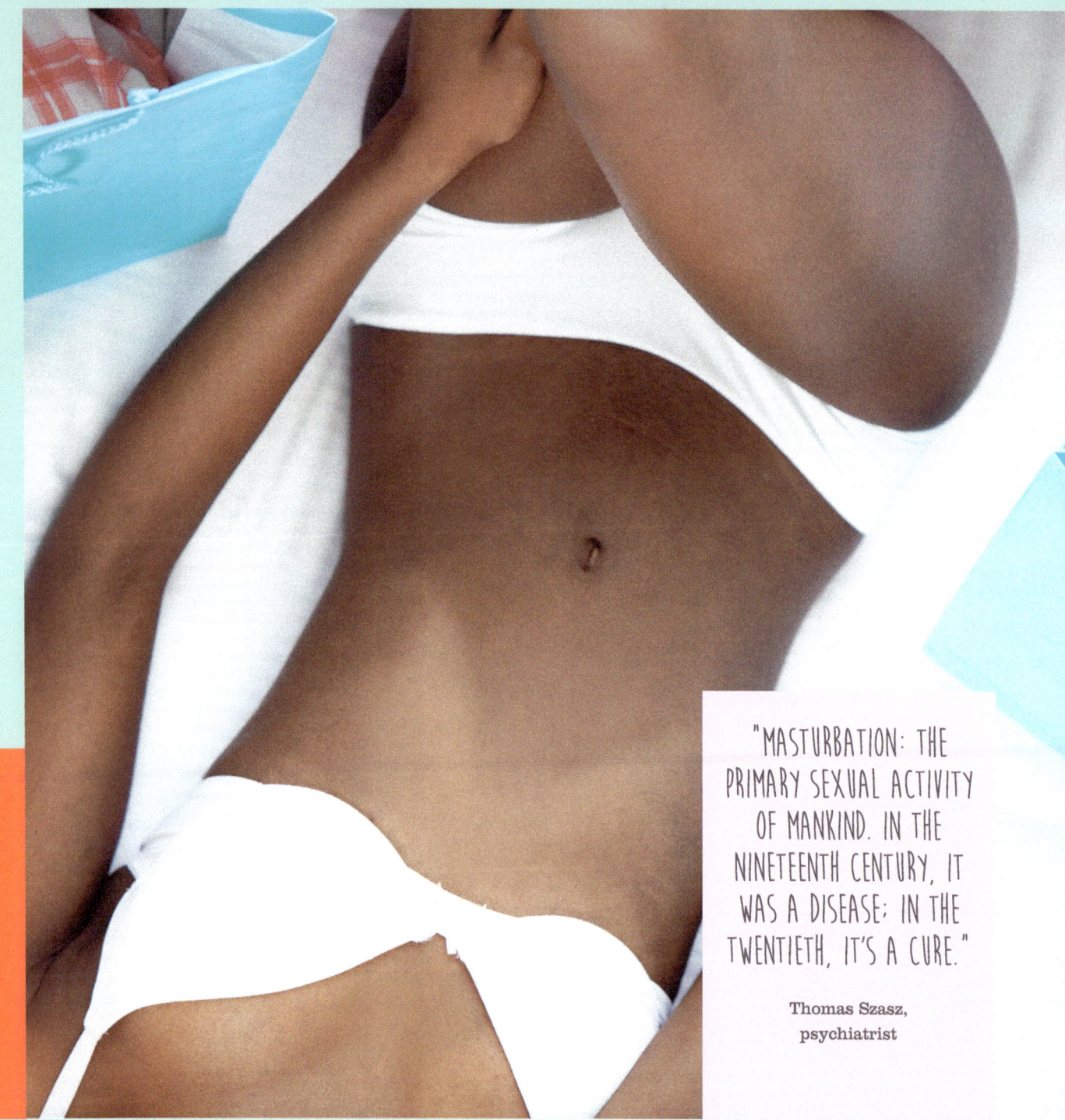

"MASTURBATION: THE PRIMARY SEXUAL ACTIVITY OF MANKIND. IN THE NINETEENTH CENTURY, IT WAS A DISEASE; IN THE TWENTIETH, IT'S A CURE."

Thomas Szasz,
psychiatrist

INTRODUCTION

Welcome to your solo sex adventure guide! If you're looking to make your sex life more varied and more fulfilling—on your own or with a partner—you've come to the right place. You may be brand new to the art of solo play, or perhaps you are an experienced connoisseur. Either way, *Sex Yourself* will help you explore the infinite possibilities of self-pleasure. The following chapters will debunk the myths that can make it tough to embrace masturbation, and will show you why (and how!) solo sex should be celebrated. You'll get an in-depth look at your erogenous anatomy, and you'll discover how to get yourself in the mood for pleasure when sex is the furthest thing from your mind. Once you're ready for some self-loving, you'll learn a whole slew of solo sex techniques, and you'll find out plenty about how sex toys and other fun accessories can make

self-pleasure even hotter. Then there's everything you need to know about orgasms: how to find them, how to make them bigger and better, and how to share them with a partner. For the grand finale, you'll find lots of ways to practice solo sex with a partner (yes, solo sex can make your partnered sex life far more exciting!).

First, let me tell you a little bit about myself. These days, I run a sexuality retail store and workshop center called Good For Her. Based in Toronto, Good For Her offers a selection of top-quality sex toys, books, DVDs, and workshops on sex and sexuality. But I grew up in a conservative household in which sex didn't exist. We never discussed it as a family, and the only intimacy I witnessed at home was my mom kissing my dad on the cheek—once. Then, when I was about six years old, I was in my room

exploring myself, trying to figure out what was going on in and around the area that pee came from. I'd never heard of a vagina, much less a clitoris. I was looking at the folds of skin between my legs—my labia—when my mom walked in on me. She didn't say anything—except to tell me to be sure to wash my hands afterward. I did, but I never explored that part of my body again as a child.

As I grew up, sex and relationships terrified me, probably because I didn't know anything about them other than what I learned from Hollywood and TV. Although I dated a little during high school, each time the intimacy moved beyond kissing, I freaked out and ran away. Finally, when I was twenty-one, I was dating someone I felt pretty comfortable with, and I decided I was ready to try sex. When we were about to take our clothes off, I stopped. "I'm terrified of your penis," I told him. "I've never seen one before." He was really patient, and after he gave me a guided tour, I decided that we could make friends, his penis and I. And we did. But when we had sex, I felt pleasure and intensity building—with no release. I didn't know what to expect, because I hadn't experimented with masturbation since my mother interrupted me fifteen years earlier. Once, my partner stopped what he was doing and asked me what I liked. "Aren't you supposed to know that?" I replied. Gently, he suggested that it might be helpful if I knew a little more about my own body, and about what brought me pleasure.

So I decided to be a good student. I tried really diligently to have an orgasm, both on my own and with my partner. No joy. I'd feel a little bit of pleasure, but no fireworks. After a while, I'd get bored and give up. After two years of focused effort, I gave up for good. I rationalized it to myself in this way: Some people are tall, others are short; some are good at math, while others are good at art; some people can orgasm, and some people can't. And you know what? I enjoyed sex, but I accepted that I wouldn't be able to have an orgasm, and I adjusted my expectations accordingly.

Several years and relationships later, my inability to orgasm got me dumped. My partner found it too stressful to have sex with me without the finale everyone expects. Well, this was a turning point for me: now my inability to orgasm was getting in the way of my relationships. So I went to a good friend for advice and asked her what I needed to do to climax. She told me I should buy the Hitachi Magic Wand, a back massager. I did. And a couple of weeks later, I had my first orgasm. Finally, I knew what everyone was talking about: I was a part of the "O" club!

As the years passed, I continued my sexual exploration: I kept buying toys and kept learning. When my sister, a United Church of Canada minister, was getting married in 1995, I bought her some fun toys to celebrate her relationship. I brought them as wrapped gifts to her bridal shower, thinking that they were a pretty typical kind of bridal shower present. Well, according to her friends—who brought wine glasses and pottery—sex toys were not regular bridal shower gifts. When they saw the toys I'd brought, my sister's friends exclaimed, "What on earth is that?" and asked, "Where do you stick it?" and "What does it do?" I answered all of their questions matter-of-factly, and they told me that because I was so comfortable talking about sex, I should start conducting workshops on the subject.

Well, that sounded like a lot of fun! My sister and her friends were my first workshop participants, and with that, my new career was born. Lots of my workshop participants told me they'd love to have access to a comfortable, professional place where they could take more workshops and buy good quality products. So I opened Good For Her, and I continued to learn from my colleagues, customers, and workshop participants. Over time, I found that so many women were struggling with masturbation, finding their erogenous zones, having orgasms with their partners, or having orgasms at all—just like I had. I enrolled in a sex therapy training program, on top of other formal and informal educational opportunities, so that I could help my customers even more—and much of this book's content is a direct result of my own experience in giving workshops and in coaching individuals and couples, as well as my own personal adventures, of course.

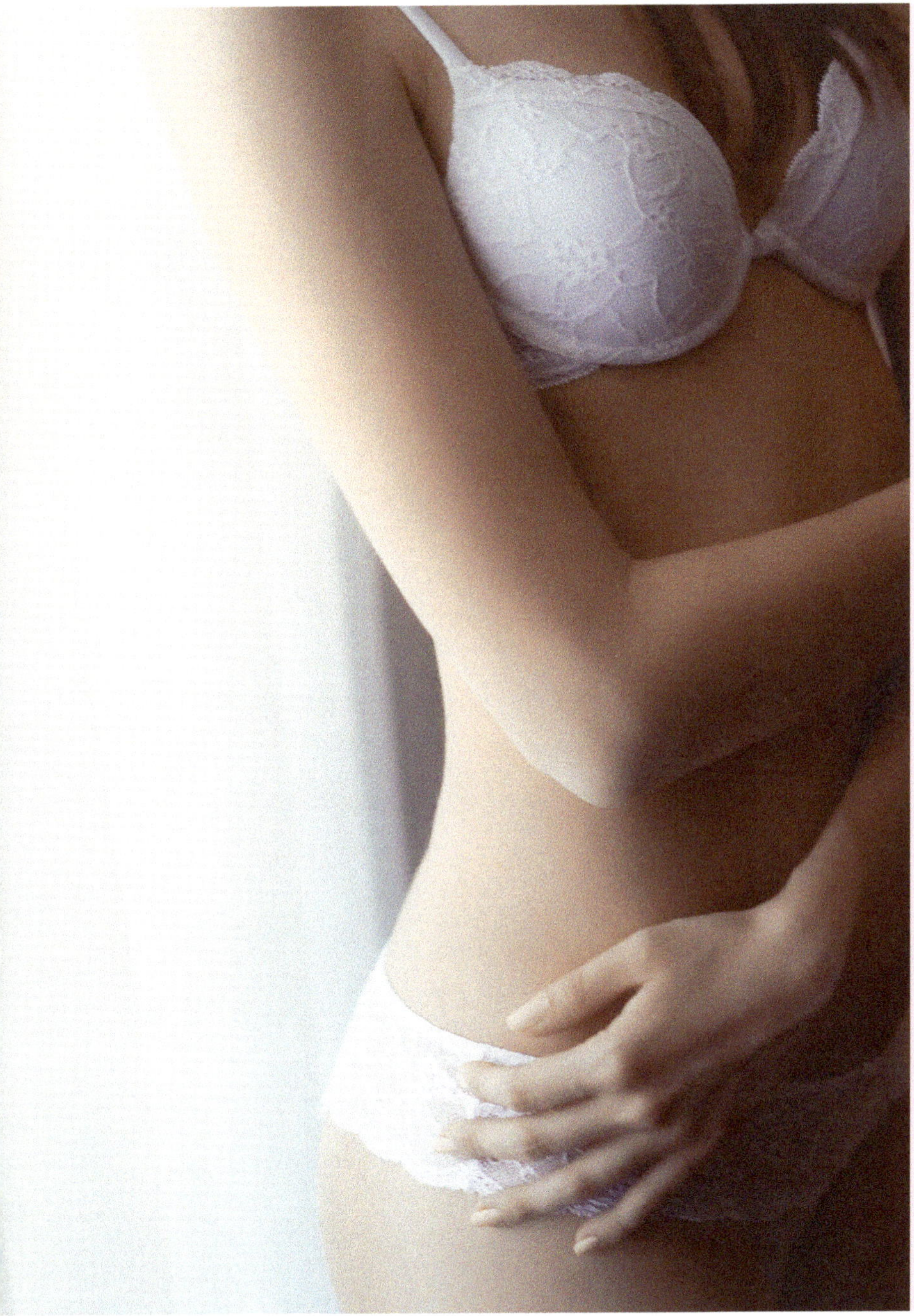

WOMEN MASTURBATE LESS OFTEN THAN MEN IN ALL AGE CATEGORIES.

And generally we all do it less frequently as we age. According to one study, about 13 percent of women between the ages of twenty and twenty-nine report having solo sex two or three times per week, compared to nearly 44 percent of men in the same age bracket. Less than 4 percent of women between the ages of fifty and fifty-nine report having solo sex that often, though nearly a quarter of their male counterparts do.

> "SEEKING SEXUAL SATISFACTION IS A BASIC DESIRE, AND MASTURBATION IS OUR FIRST NATURAL SEXUAL ACTIVITY. IT'S THE WAY WE DISCOVER OUR EROTICISM, THE WAY WE LEARN TO RESPOND SEXUALLY, THE WAY WE LEARN TO LOVE OURSELVES AND TO BUILD SELF-ESTEEM."
>
> Betty Dodson, author and sex educator

WHO ARE YOU?

Maybe you're reading this book because you're curious and want to learn more about your body and how it works. Or maybe you don't really enjoy sex, and you want to figure out how to make it (more) pleasurable. Perhaps you haven't been able to orgasm (yet!) and a friend or therapist suggested reading a book on masturbation. Or perhaps your partner is experiencing some of these concerns. Whatever your goals are, *Sex Yourself* is here to help.

A (VERY) BRIEF HISTORY OF MASTURBATION

Although many historians believe that prehistoric peoples had positive attitudes toward solo sex, as evidenced by cave paintings and figurines, masturbation tends to get a bad rap in contemporary Western culture. And that's putting it mildly. In fact, the word itself is laden with negative connotations: Etymologically, the word

GUILT IS COMMON.

At least one study showed that approximately 50 percent of women and 50 percent of men who masturbate feel guilty about it.

MASTURBATION WAS DECLARED A NORMAL ACTIVITY BY THE AMERICAN MEDICAL ASSOCIATION IN 1972.

*masturbatio*n derives from the Latin words *manus* ("hand") and *stuprare* ("to defile oneself"). "Defiling oneself with the hand"—is it really so surprising that self-pleasure comes with so much baggage attached? Whether you grew up in a sex-positive household or not, you're probably aware that there's a sort of pejorative aura surrounding solo sex, especially for girls and women. Implicitly or explicitly, girls are often taught that masturbating makes them "dirty," "impure," "selfish," or even "slutty." In fact, in nineteenth-century Europe, clitoridectomies, or the removal of women's clitorises, were performed in order to stop girls and women from masturbating. Doctors claimed that female masturbation induced conditions such as hysteria, spinal irritation, epilepsy, mental disability, mania, and even death.

Of course, these theories have long since been disproved, and, in recent years, solo sex has come out of the closet in a big way. It's been endorsed by many health professionals as a healthy activity, and in 2009, several European nations introduced progressive materials encouraging teens to masturbate. One UK pamphlet explained that, like the proverbial apple, "an orgasm a day keeps the doctor away," emphasizing the importance of masturbation as part of a healthy lifestyle, just like exercising and eating your vegetables. Many progressive organizations around the world, such as Planned Parenthood, also endorse solo sex as a reliable, healthy, respectable form of sexual self-expression. So, go ahead and celebrate the beauty of solo sex: It's a wonderful way to maintain good physical and mental health, and to enjoy your own unique, individual, beautiful body. Let's get started!

A NOTE ABOUT TERMINOLOGY

Masturbation is the technical term for erotic self-stimulation. But it's not a very sexy word, and it may even carry a lot of negative connotations for many of us. So, throughout this book, I use "masturbation," "solo sex," and "self-pleasure" interchangeably. They all mean exactly the same thing: taking pleasure into your own hands.

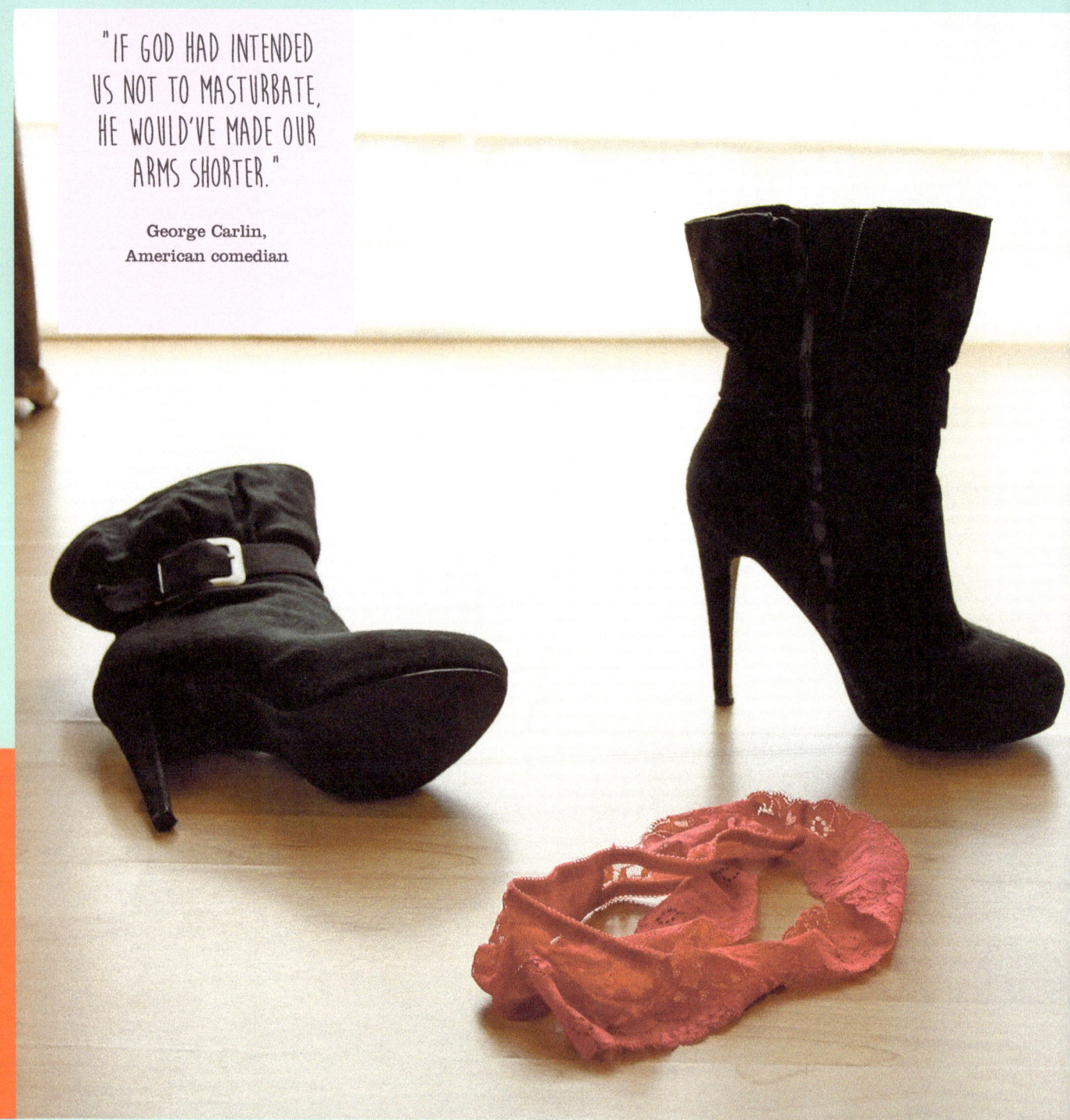

"IF GOD HAD INTENDED US NOT TO MASTURBATE, HE WOULD'VE MADE OUR ARMS SHORTER."

George Carlin,
American comedian

1

HEALTHY SOLO SEX

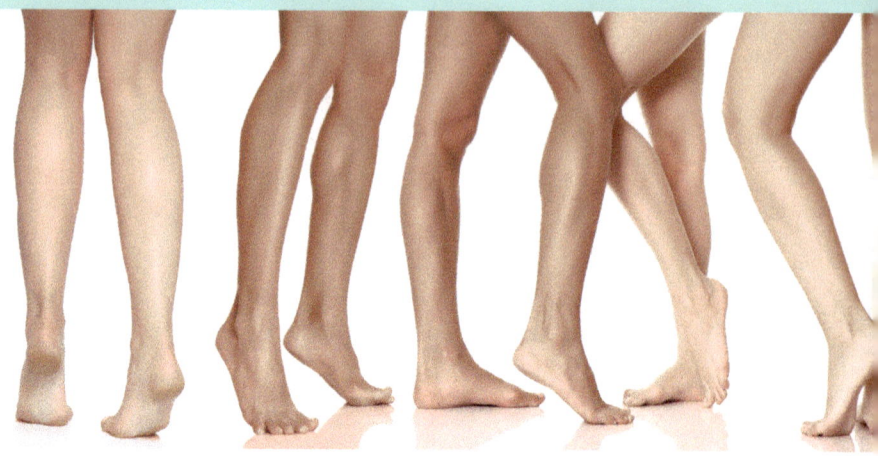

As children and teenagers, many of us weren't given much, if any, information about sex. Even though the twentieth and twenty-first centuries have witnessed major developments in technology and education, sex is still a taboo subject in many households. That means lots of young people, especially girls and young women, aren't comfortable or confident talking about it, and they end up with a jumble of incorrect information garnered from popular culture about their bodies and their sexuality—plus a barrage of shame-filled messages about sexual pleasure, partner sex, and solo play. And although sex education is part of the curriculum in most schools, it's usually far from perfect. Even the best sex education programs can't cover everything, and they're often complicated or limited by the personal values each teacher holds, and by her or his level of comfort with the subject. What all this boils down to is, most of us have a thing or two to learn when it comes to sex—especially solo sex. After all, teachers may have taught you the basics of anatomy in school, but I bet you've never taken a class on how to masturbate!

That's where *Sex Yourself* comes in. This book will give you all the tools and information you need to have sensational solo sex, either alone or with a partner. In the coming pages (no pun intended!), you'll learn things you didn't know that you didn't know. You'll find out why masturbation is great for your health: It helps improve sleep quality, decreases stress levels, prevents depression, and lots more. It can also provide powerful pain relief, increase your sexual confidence, and boost your immune system. In the process, you'll learn new masturbation techniques that'll shake up your routine—and you'll teach yourself to achieve better orgasms, enhancing both solo sex and sex with a partner.

First things first, though: It's time to tackle some of the most common misconceptions about masturbation. In this chapter, I'll show you why masturbation can boost your psychological and physical health, and how it can make partner sex that much hotter.

An online survey of 178 women by HealthyStrokes.com in 2003 found that 41 percent of women found solo sex "more fun" than intercourse.

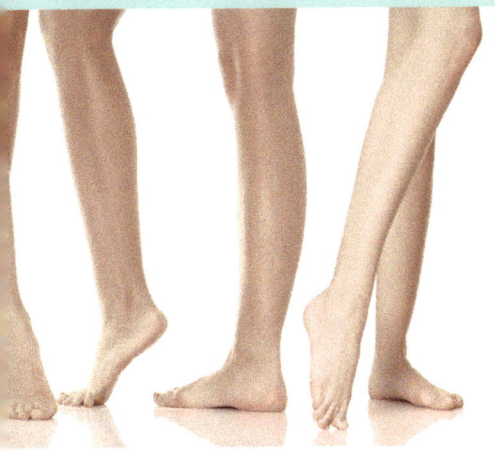

LET'S TALK ABOUT SEX

I'm often asked whether solo sex counts as "real" sex. The answer is a resounding *yes!*

Sexual pleasure comes in many forms, and the truth is, it can be enjoyed by one person, two people, or more than two people at a time. See, when it comes to pleasure, your body doesn't discriminate: pleasure is pleasure, whether it's provided by toys, fingers, hands, or other parts of the body. Of course, the energy and emotions that exist between people do make a difference in the way a person responds to touch. But, at the end of the day, the same touch in the same spot in the same way is interpreted by our nerve endings as pleasure—regardless of who's providing the entertainment.

So, if I'm having sex with myself, does that mean I'm cheating on my partner? No way. First and foremost, your body belongs to you, and that means you're already in a relationship with yourself, whether you choose to engage with it sexually or not. When you're in a sexual relationship with another person or persons, your self-pleasure doesn't compete or interfere with those relationship(s). Far from it, in fact: Lots of people find that, if anything, solo sex actually enhances partner sex.

In my experience, some people feel that sexual pleasure should be about sharing with someone else, and that it's more "natural" and less selfish to focus on their partner's pleasure. Sure, sharing a sexual experience with a partner or partners can be wonderful—but when it comes to pleasure, there's no such thing as right or wrong. As long as you're not harming yourself or others, there's no reason why you shouldn't take pleasure in your own sexuality, just as you might

WHAT IS SEX?

The word *sex* is often used as shorthand for the term "sexual intercourse," which usually refers to inserting a penis into a vagina. But sex can be so much more than that—and that's part of what makes it so exciting! It's not necessarily limited to certain parts of the body (or to any parts of the body), and it can involve any combination of penises, vaginas, nipples, butts, or clitorises. For example, a person may have a vagina, but she might only want to have her clitoris touched. And that's just the beginning: oral sex, anal sex, kinky sex, sex alone, phone sex, and sex with two or more people are also forms of sex. In this book, I use the term *sex* to mean any expressions or activities that are intended to arouse yourself and/or a partner or partners.

take pleasure in food, fashion, or massage. In fact, studies show that people who masturbate regularly tend to be more confident lovers, and are more likely to be sexually satisfied with their partners. If you can't do it for yourself at first, that's okay: Think of it as a way to develop a better sexual relationship with your partner!

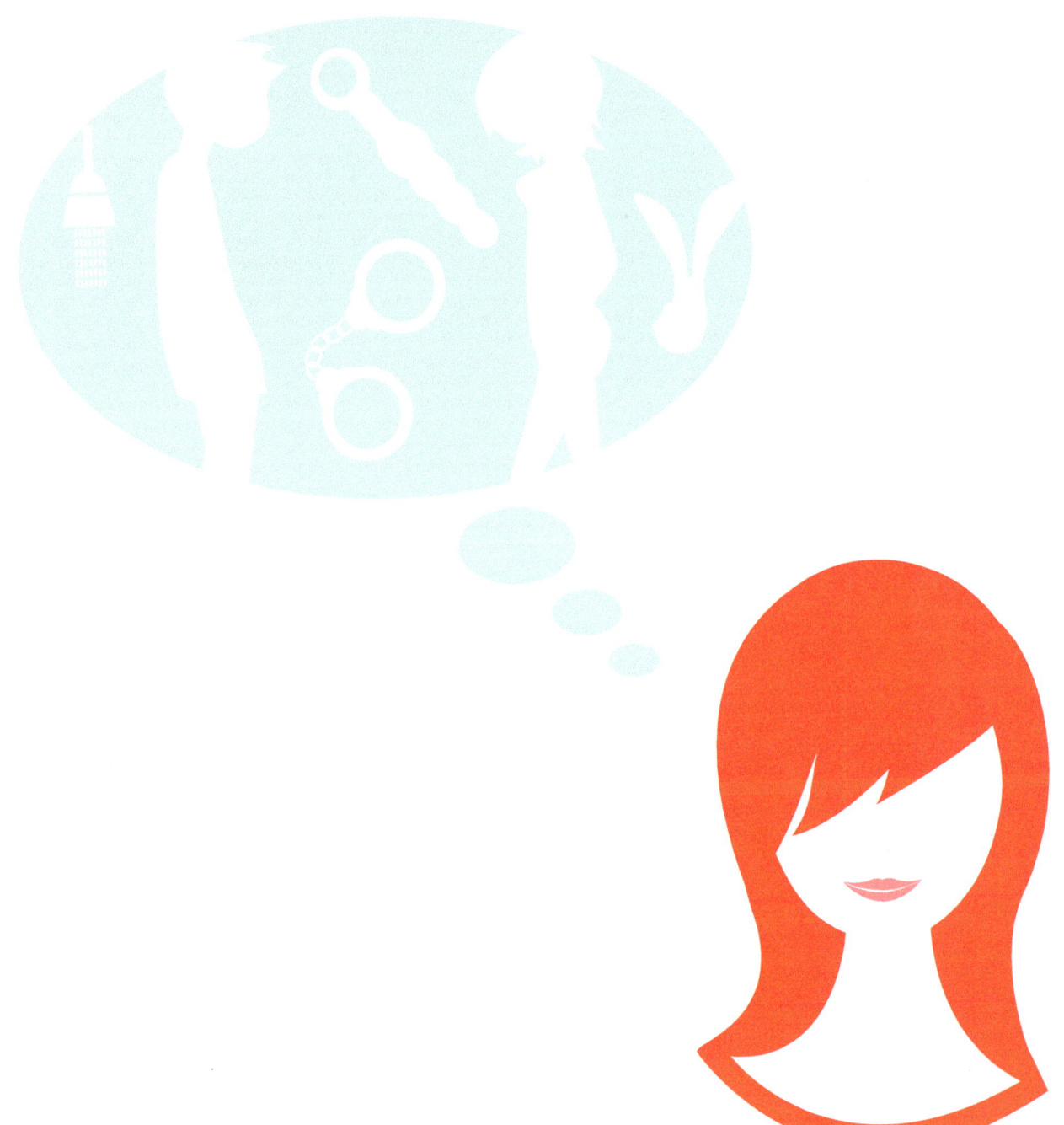

MASTURBATION CAN HELP YOU LEARN TO ORGASM.

One study found that 90 percent of those who followed a masturbation program were able to learn to orgasm through solo pleasure, 85 percent from direct stimulation by their partner, and 40 percent from intercourse!

Just how good can masturbation be, though? Can it ever be as good as partner sex? Absolutely! In fact, some folks swear that solo sex is even better than partner sex, because you know your own body more intuitively and can respond to your own desire faster and more accurately than any partner could. While it's true that the chemistry, energy, and emotions that are sparked by sex with a partner aren't a part of solo sex, all it takes is a little imagination to conjure them up. By connecting with yourself and tuning in to your own moods and emotions, you can channel the chemistry and energy aroused by a current, former, or fantasy partner during sex with yourself. It's impossible to overestimate the power of self-connection; it's truly the key to hot solo sex. (Looking for strategies to help you fire up your solo sex routine? You'll find plenty of inspiration in chapter 6.)

What's more, studies have shown that a great sexual relationship with yourself can mean a better sexual relationship with your partner or partners. People who engage in self-pleasure tend to be more confident because they know their own bodies well and are more comfortable with them. And confidence is definitely sexy. So ignore the messages sent by the media! Masturbation isn't for losers who can't find a partner. In fact, the opposite is true: a 1994 study found that 45 percent of women who were living with a partner still engaged in solo sex (as did 85 percent of men). Plus, masturbation is an ongoing learning experience. It's healthy to keep those juices flowing—both literally and figuratively—because it's a great way to figure out what turns you on, to discover new things about your own body, and to honor your relationship with yourself. And, of course, sharing your sexual self-knowledge with your partner can make sex *à deux* that much hotter.

MORE SOLO SEX EQUALS MORE PARTNER SEX.

Several studies indicate that the more a person with a partner masturbates, the more likely she or he is to engage in partner sex. Interestingly, the same studies show that gay men and lesbian women masturbate more regularly than their straight counterparts.

Finally, how much is too much? Can solo sex be addictive? Well, you can overdo or obsess about nearly anything—including exercise and eating well—and that can get in the way of other areas of your life, such as your career or your relationships. As long as your solo sex life is balanced and doesn't interfere with your relationships, your work life, or your health, then go ahead and celebrate it!

LOVE YOURSELF

At least one study has demonstrated that the more frequently a woman masturbates, the more positive her body image tends to be.

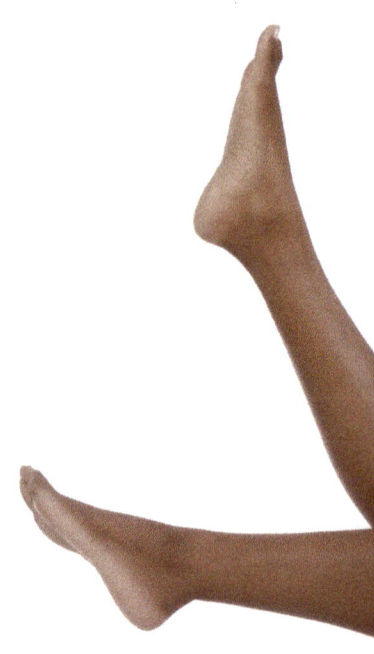

GETTING PHYSICAL

Although the health benefits of masturbation have been proven by dozens of scientific studies, rumors about its detrimental health effects have run rampant for generations. In the past, many religious communities claimed that solo sex causes everything from baldness and blindness to unwanted hair growth and mental health illnesses to discourage people from masturbating. These views were often based on interpretations of religious texts that frowned upon any kind of sexual activity that didn't have procreation as its main goal—including solo sex. Over the years—and especially in the late nineteenth and early twentieth centuries—hundreds of "anti-masturbation" products were developed: everything from breakfast cereal to published pamphlets to scary-looking electric belts that promised to reduce the wearers' urge to masturbate. But the medical community disproved such theories long ago, and today, most medical professionals advocate solo sex as a healthy habit for both body and mind.

It's still important to be mindful of your health when you're enjoying solo sex. Like any other activity, sex, whether solo or partnered, has its risks. Happily, masturbation rarely places you at risk for sexually transmitted infections (STIs). There's one exception to this, though, and that's sharing sex toys with a partner who has an STI such as the human papilloma virus, because HPV may still be able to survive even on silicone toys up to twenty-four hours after they've been cleaned. Otherwise, simply using lubricant can prevent redness or soreness. It can make solo sex more pleasurable by helping fingers and toys glide in and out more easily, in the same way that oil is useful when you're getting or giving a massage. And when it comes to toys, always choose wisely: using the right toys for vaginal or anal insertion will prevent them from getting lost inside you, and from

MASTURBATION CAN HELP YOU FALL ASLEEP.

While no formal studies have proven it (yet), an informal survey in 2010 on CureTogether.com found that masturbation is 50 percent effective for treating insomnia, because orgasm floods the brain with endorphins and oxytocin, the "feel-good" hormone. (And—surprise, surprise—it's a relatively popular option.) Why not try it the next time you find yourself counting sheep?

harming sensitive internal linings. (Speaking of which, if you've used sex toys anally, be sure to sterilize them before you use them vaginally so you won't contract bacterial infections.) Finally, just as you'd choose eco-friendly body care products whenever possible, respect your body and the planet by going for eco-friendly toys and lubricants. (Chapter 5 will help you select the sexual products that are best—and safest—for you.)

FINDING ME-TIME

Life gets busy, and most of us have a lot of pressing responsibilities that require our time and attention. Understandably, you might not feel you've got the extra energy and headspace to invest in this part of your life after you've raced home from work, walked the dog, cooked for the kids, exercised, cleaned the house, volunteered for the community, finished your schoolwork, and spent time with your partner, family, or friends. (Whew!) Try looking at it this way, though: Experimenting with self-pleasure doesn't have to take hours, and it's a fun, healthy activity—not another boring chore. That might help motivate you to squeeze a little you-time into your busy day.

SOLO PLEASURE BOOSTS YOUR SELF-ESTEEM.

A 2009 study showed that women with low self-esteem and poor body image are able to increase their self-esteem through masturbation, which enables them to learn more about their bodies.

Need a few more reasons to have solo sex? Here's why you should get busy with yourself—right now! Masturbation can:

» Help you fall asleep quickly, sleep soundly, and reduce insomnia

» Boost your immune system to help you fight infection

» Increase your sexual confidence and improve your mood and overall self-esteem

» Decrease stress levels, assist in combating high blood pressure, prevent depression, and lower the risk of type 2 diabetes

» Combat menstrual pain and reduce chronic back pain and migraines

» Help prevent cervical infections and urinary tract infections (UTIs)

» Increase pelvic floor strength, leading to better sex and less incontinence

» Stimulate your brain, preventing the onset of dementia

» Get your blood pumping

Solo sex is a safe, rewarding, satisfying way to explore your sexuality, tune in to your own body, and figure out what feels good for you. It's also fabulous for your mental and physical health, and it can help you become a more confident lover. So what are you waiting for? Read on for an in-depth look at your erotic anatomy, and find out how to explore your own erogenous zones. Incredible solo sex is just a few pages away.

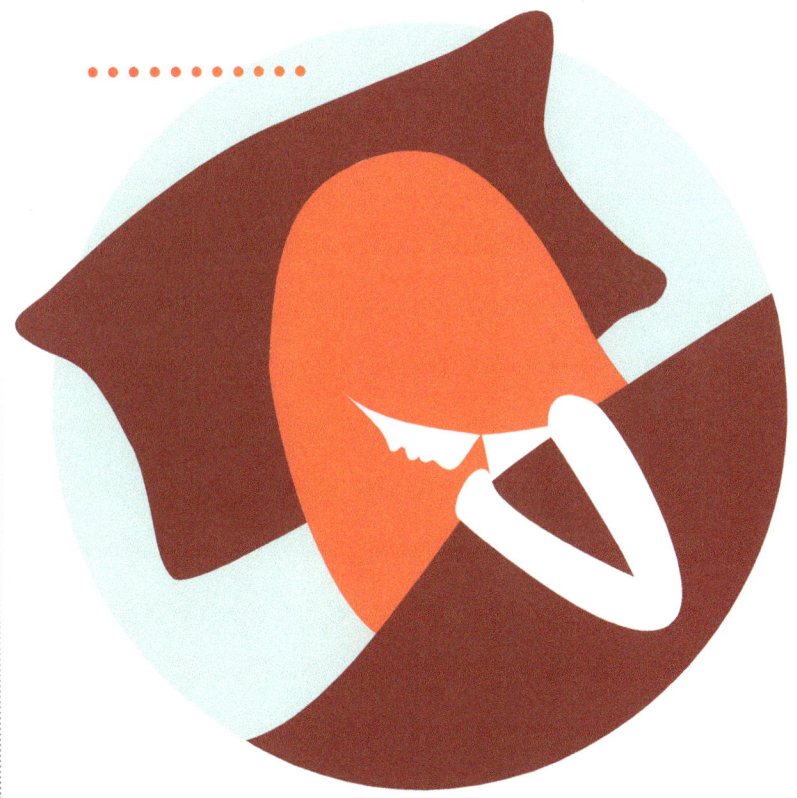

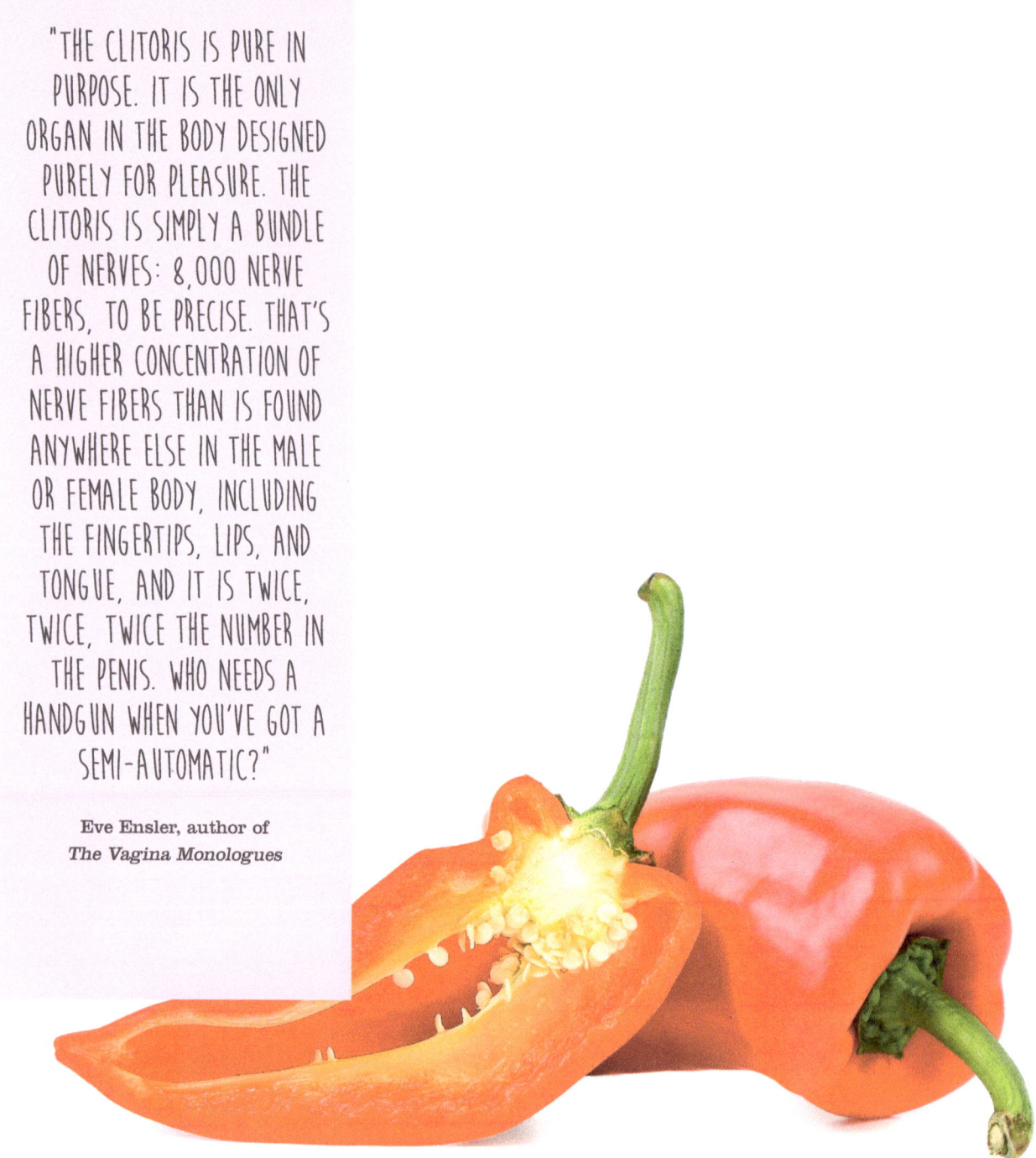

"THE CLITORIS IS PURE IN PURPOSE. IT IS THE ONLY ORGAN IN THE BODY DESIGNED PURELY FOR PLEASURE. THE CLITORIS IS SIMPLY A BUNDLE OF NERVES: 8,000 NERVE FIBERS, TO BE PRECISE. THAT'S A HIGHER CONCENTRATION OF NERVE FIBERS THAN IS FOUND ANYWHERE ELSE IN THE MALE OR FEMALE BODY, INCLUDING THE FINGERTIPS, LIPS, AND TONGUE, AND IT IS TWICE, TWICE, TWICE THE NUMBER IN THE PENIS. WHO NEEDS A HANDGUN WHEN YOU'VE GOT A SEMI-AUTOMATIC?"

Eve Ensler, author of
The Vagina Monologues

2

ANATOMY, HOT SPOTS, AND EROGENOUS ZONES

This is the story most of us were told as kids: Boys have penises and girls have vaginas. And when sex happens, it's supposed to work like a puzzle, or like one of those flat-packed bookshelves that are supposed to be so easy to assemble: Insert penis A into vagina B. (Yawn.) But the fact is, there's so much more to sexual pleasure. Sure, sex *can* involve a penis and a vagina–but it doesn't have to revolve completely around them. Sex can mean one vagina or one penis (as in solo sex), or it can mean two vaginas, or two penises, or one or more of each. Pleasure is truly a movable feast, and there are infinite ways to experience it–even when you're getting busy with yourself.

Because the penis-and-vagina model has been drilled into us for so long, it's no wonder that so many women aren't down with their own erotic anatomy. You may have heard of that magic button called the clitoris–but what's a G-spot, and does it really exist? Is there such a thing as female ejaculation? Do women actually enjoy anal sex? How can I have an orgasm from vaginal stimulation? This book will tackle all these questions, and plenty more. Great sex–with yourself or a partner–is something you can learn, and learning is half the fun!

SEX IS A SKILL

Wait a minute. What's there to learn about masturbation? It's pretty straightforward, isn't it? You stick your hand down under your underwear, do your thing, and *voilà!* –the earth shakes and you're done. If pop culture, porn, and Hollywood are to be believed, all women can rock their own bodies whenever

VULVA VS. VAGINA?

The word *vagina* is commonly used to refer to women's genitals in general. But your vagina is actually a specific part of your anatomy: it's the internal passage that extends from your vulva to your cervix. The external part of your genital area is called the vulva. Together, the vulva and vagina make up the majority of a woman's erogenous pleasure zones.

they want to, and with just about any kind of stimulation Down There. Well, the fact is, movies and porn usually portray fantasies, not realistic sexual experiences. So if we really want to learn about sex and pleasure, we need other resources–ones that are truthful, accurate, and woman-friendly.

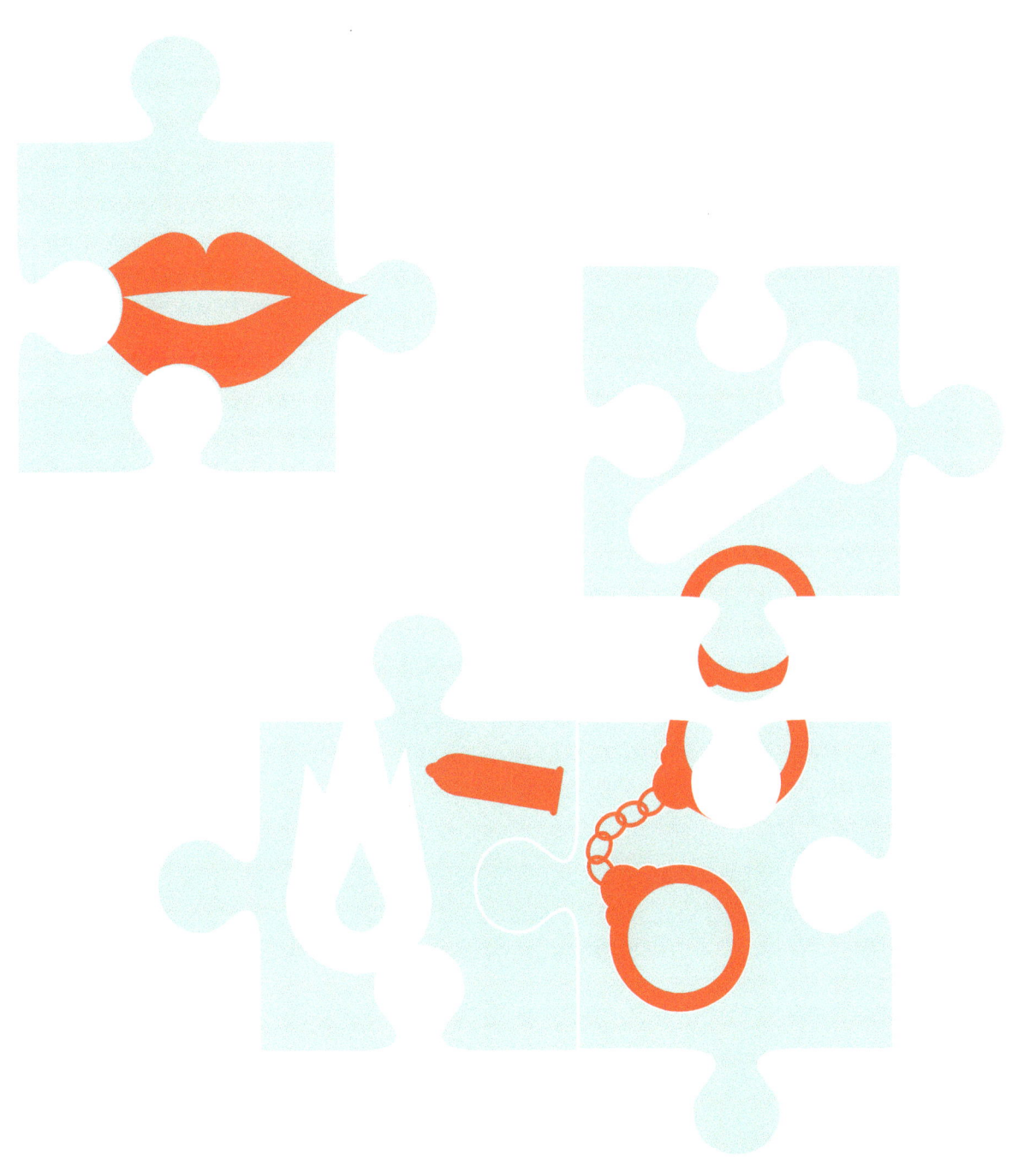

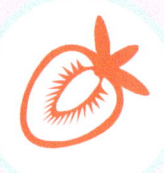

PUSSY PRAISE

There's no lack of alternative names or nicknames knocking around for vulvas and vaginas. Here are just a few of the more positive ones: beaver, cooch, kitty, love cave, madame, muffin, poonani, pussy, twat, vajayjay. What do you call yours?

Knowing how to have sex isn't something you're born with. It's a skill, and like anything else, the more you learn, the more satisfying it becomes. Anyone can kick a ball around a soccer field; learning the techniques and strategies of the game is what makes you a stronger player. Of course, there's no law that says you *have* to hone your skills. You *could* just keep having sex the way you always have and hope for the best—but if you choose that path, sex may become more boring and less pleasurable, and you might eventually lose interest in it altogether. Alternatively, you could spend time learning about your beautiful, unique body, explore new sexual options and sensations, and make great sex a lifelong habit. Which path would you choose?

All this is to show you just how important solo sex is. Not only it is a pleasurable type of sex in its own right, but it's also a valuable skill. Masturbation might seem "easier" than partner sex because you're focusing on your own body, not another person's—but the reality is, it's not always second nature. That's because we're so often discouraged from thinking of solo pleasure as a respectable, natural type of self-expression, and because so many of us simply weren't taught enough about our bodies. The result? Solo play seems like a bit of a mystery. Some folks are lucky, and discover their erogenous zones easily or even by accident—and are rewarded with mind-blowing multiple orgasms. That experience is relatively rare, but if you happen to be one of those lucky folks, good for you! Hopefully, you'll still be interested in exploring new aspects of solo pleasure; after all, just because you're already a great cook doesn't mean you can't sample new cuisines and learn a few new kitchen tricks. There's always more to learn about our bodies and how they work.

BATTLE OF THE SEXES

So where do you start? It's easy to say "Go explore!" but most women need a little more guidance than that—not least because most of the erogenous zones on our bodies are located either beneath the skin or inside the vagina and can't easily be seen. Simply looking at yourself won't give you much of an idea about where, or how, to start. And, unlike men, we don't generally touch most of those areas while engaging in nonsexual activities like using the toilet, showering, or getting dressed. If we do discover what we enjoy during partner sex, we rarely stop our partners to ask, "Can you show me where you're touching me and how you're doing it?" Instead, we usually carry on with the pleasure at hand and hope we get to feel it again the next time around. But that's far from a perfect solution: Women often describe amazing sexual experiences that they've enjoyed once and have been trying to recapture ever since. And knowing what your body is capable of but feeling as if it's beyond your reach can be terribly frustrating. There's a remedy, though: a little self-knowledge.

It's completely okay if you're not sure where to start. It's not just you. Women often succumb to the double standard that surrounds masturbation—the one that tells us that it's okay for boys to masturbate because "boys will be boys," but "good girls" don't touch themselves. When women do begin to masturbate, they usually do so later than men: women generally start in their twenties, while most boys begin before the age of ten. Society tells us that men "can't help themselves" and that it's "natural" for them, with their higher libidos, to enjoy their penises solo. Men are even sometimes encouraged to do it, as a way to take care of their own needs when they're single, or when their partner isn't interested or available. Women, on the other hand, struggle to accept that it's natural, normal, healthy, and acceptable for them to touch and pleasure themselves, too.

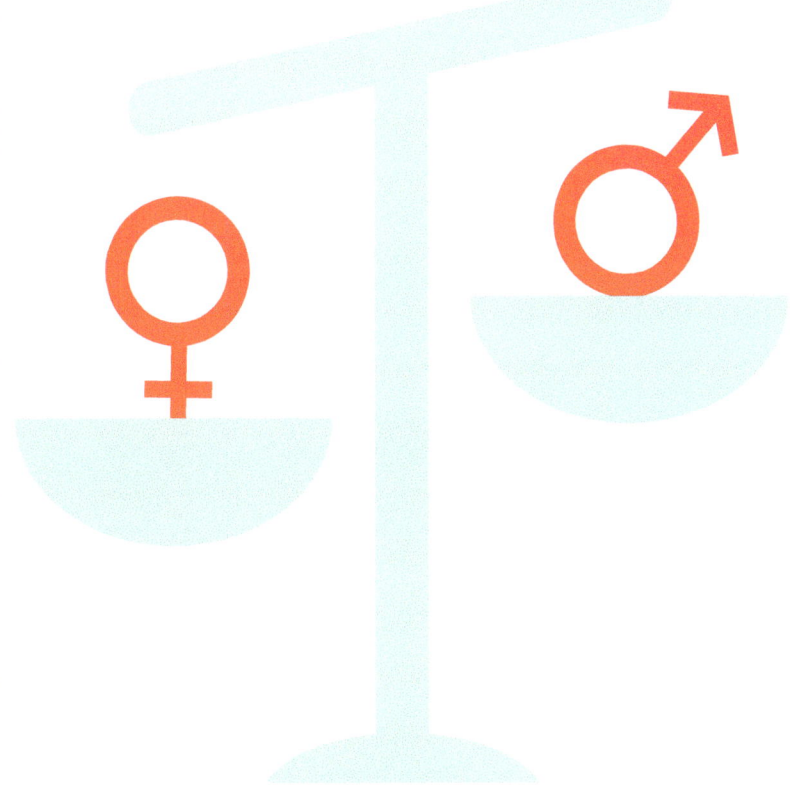

GENDER GAP

More boys (75 percent) than girls (45 percent) masturbate at age sixteen to seventeen. They also do it more often: 50 percent of boys engage in solo sex at least twice a week, compared to 23 percent of girls.

What's more, women's erotic network of nerve endings, erogenous zones, and pleasure options is more complicated than men's: neuronal pathways in women are much more intricate and complex. While erotic responses in men are generally more straightforward and simple, sources of arousal and pleasure in women are difficult to pinpoint. Plus, erogenous zones often differ from woman to woman. What men find pleasurable is relatively (but not completely) consistent—but what works for one woman rarely works for another. When it comes to erotic preferences, each woman is unique. And even if two women share a common erogenous zone, the way in which they enjoy its stimulation can vary. For example, some women can tolerate only gentle touch on the clitoris, while others crave intense, jackhammer pressure—and some women don't enjoy clitoral stimulation at all. As you explore your erogenous zones, you'll figure out what feels good to you and how you like it. You'll learn whether you like intense or gentle pressure, fast or slow strokes, long or short movements, direct pressure or circular motions. You'll also find that what you like might change as your sexual encounter progresses: at the beginning of arousal, after intense stimulation, or at the edge of orgasm. Each woman develops her own individual preferences, which can also vary from day to day.

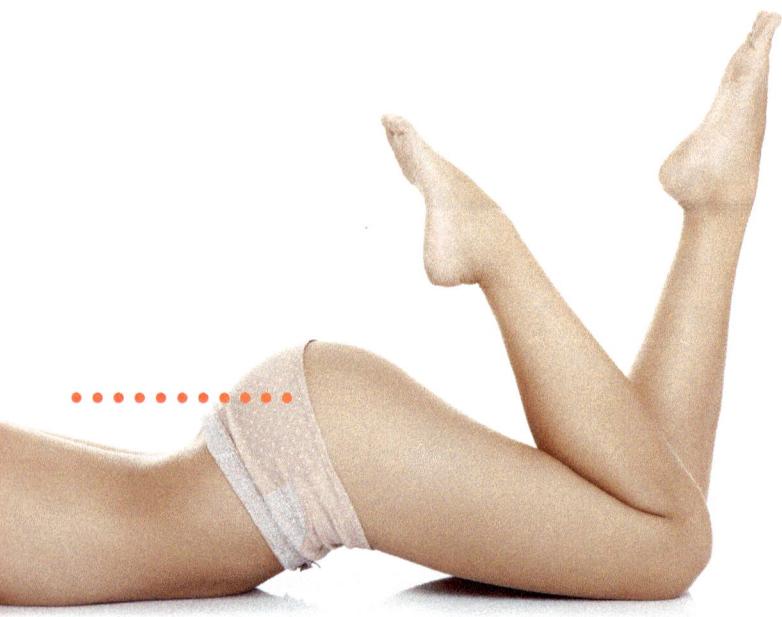

NON-GENITAL EROGENOUS ZONES

Start by exploring your not-so-obvious erogenous zones. These areas of your body are key to your overall sexual arousal. You'll find that pretty much any part of your body that has skin will be responsive to touch—even your eyelids! So go ahead and experiment. Try soft, long strokes or light strokes that barely graze the hairs of your skin. Play around with textures, stimulating your skin with a silky scarf in contrast with your nails. (See chapter 5 for more ideas.) Let your fingers dance gently—as if you were playing the piano without heavy pressure—on various parts of your body. You can also try squeezing, jiggling, rubbing in circles, using a firm touch lubricated by massage oil or lotion, gentle tapping, firm slapping, you name it. Of course, some styles of touch make more sense for some areas than others, and you'll find that you'll prefer some types of touch to others, depending on your level of arousal. Here are some great ways to pleasure your erogenous zones:

WHAT IS AN EROGENOUS ZONE?

Etymologically, *erogenous* means "love-producing," so erogenous zones are literally love-producing areas. These areas of your body have a heightened sensitivity to touch, and they often respond to (desired) touch with arousal or even orgasm. Some erogenous zones, such as the clitoris or penis, are pretty universal: Most people become aroused when they're stimulated, and stimulation usually produces a more intense response. Other erogenous zones, such as the inner arm or the scalp, are subtler, and touching them produces varied levels of arousal. And, most importantly, there's no such thing as one-size-fits-all. No single "map" of one body's erogenous zones will fit another because each person has her own preferences.

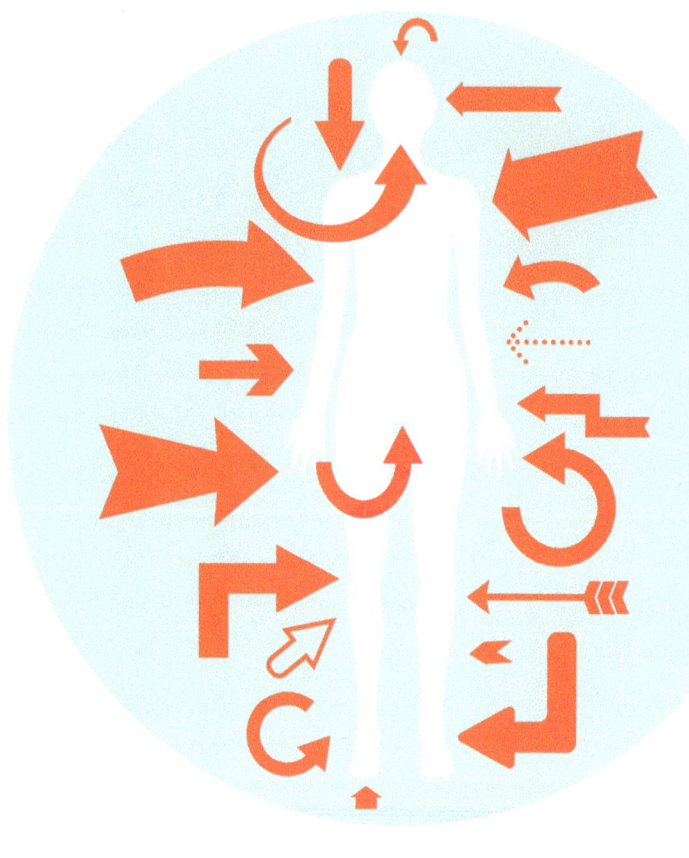

» **SCALP AND HEAD:** Use the pads of your fingers or your fingernails to massage or gently scratch your scalp.

» **EARLOBES:** Roll the lobe between your thumb and index finger, in the same way you'd roll a pen between your fingers.

» **NECK:** The neck is considered to be the most universal erogenous zone for women, and responds well to gentle touch.

» **SHOULDERS AND UPPER BACK AND CHEST:** A little self-massage or a few long, gentle strokes will go a long way.

» **SIDES OF YOUR BODY:** Run your fingers over the skin that covers your ribs: this area's super-sensual.

» **BREASTS (NIPPLE, AREOLA, UNDERSIDE, SIDES, AND TOP OF BREAST):** For some women, breast play is essential for arousal; for others, it's not much more exciting than stimulating the elbow.

» **INNER ARM, BOTH UPPER AND LOWER:** Slowly run the pads of your fingers up and down the sensitive skin of your inner arms.

» **ARMPIT:** Stroke it with your fingertips—especially after a bath or shower.

» PALM, FINGERS, AND BACK OF THE HAND: They may not be as sensitive as, say, your neck or breasts, but they love a little attention. Run the tip of one finger around the skin on your other hand, from knuckle to nail to palm, then repeat the process with the edge of your fingernail.

» LOWER ABDOMEN: The soft skin of your lower belly loves to be touched—by any part of the hand, in just about any way.

» INNER THIGHS: Graze the skin or hair on your inner thighs lightly with a finger or two—it's incredibly arousing.

» BUTT CHEEKS: They often like it rough-and-tumble, so use broad, firm strokes on them!

» CRACK OF THE BUTT: Don't use too much pressure here, because the magic crack responds well to anything that glides up and down it gently.

» BACK OF THE CALF: Massage it gently, or if you find that too ticklish, stroke the skin with the palm of your hand or your fingertips.

» TOES AND FEET: Like your hands, these guys love attention. Firm pressure, gentle pressure, whatever takes your fancy; you can't go wrong. Add a little lotion for glide, and don't forget the toes!

"DOWN THERE"

As children, we were probably presented with the "reproductive" version of sexuality by parents and teachers: girls have vaginas, and boys have penises. As I mentioned at the beginning of this chapter, it's hardly that simple, and this polarized approach to sexuality shortchanges girls and boys alike when they start to explore their erotic potential. Many girls and women feel disappointed by their first sexual experiences because they've been led to believe that the vagina is the ultimate—or even the only—erogenous zone they have. Even when we finally discover that the clitoris is a tremendously responsive erogenous zone, it's likely that we're still missing out on huge territories of our erotic geography and all the pleasurable possibilities that come with them.

It's time to get the lay of the land. I'm going to take you on a guided tour of the multiple erogenous options our bodies offer. Grab a mirror, and use it to help you get a good look at your body as we go along. You might be surprised that what you see is not what you thought it looked like, or how you remembered it to be. Also, know that every person's body is different. Your vulva is unique in the same way that your face is unique, even though we all have two eyes, a nose, and a mouth. Vulvas come in different shapes, sizes, and colors, so appreciate the uniqueness of your own vulva instead of comparing it to what you've seen in the media or on other people, or to how you imagine a vulva should look. The wonderful truth is, no one else looks quite like you! If you don't believe me, check out *I'll Show You Mine* by Wrenna Robertson, a beautiful book that showcases the diversity of women's vulvas.

Experiment with different types of touch on different areas of your body, and pay attention to the sensations. It's okay if some areas don't feel particularly good when touched, or if other areas don't feel good to the touch unless you're aroused.

VULVA

MONS PUBIS: This is the fleshy area that's located on top of your pubic bone. After puberty, it gets thicker and fatter, and becomes covered with hair.

OUTER LIPS/LABIA: The outer lips, or labia, are large, fleshy folds of skin that enclose the rest of the vulva. They're more easily visible when you're standing in front of a mirror, because they generally flatten out when you spread your legs. The outer lips begin at the mons and then separate, ending at the perineum. Like the mons pubis, they're naturally covered with hair.

ON THE SURFACE

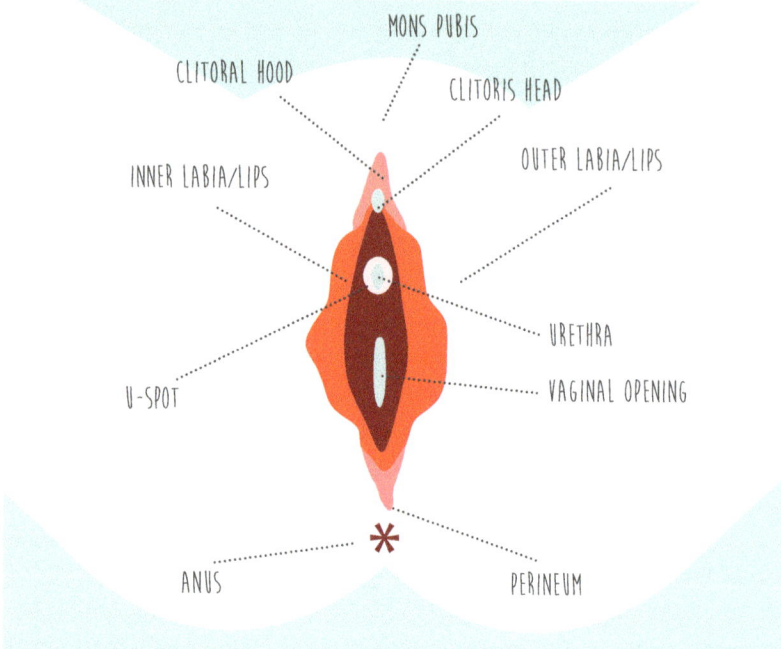

MONS PUBIS
CLITORAL HOOD
CLITORIS HEAD
OUTER LABIA/LIPS
INNER LABIA/LIPS
URETHRA
VAGINAL OPENING
U-SPOT
ANUS
PERINEUM

INNER LIPS/LABIA: These are two smaller folds of skin within the outer lips, and they vary in size, shape, and color. If you're lucky enough to have larger labia, you can grab onto them for extra sensation during solo sex. Because the inner labia extend up and around (toward the mons pubis) to form the **CLITORAL HOOD**, stimulation of the lips indirectly and gently rubs the shaft and head of the clitoris.

URETHRAL OPENING: This is the opening from which urine—and, for some women, female ejaculate—comes. It's a separate opening from the vagina,

although that's not always easy to tell: the urethral opening can be difficult to see, and it's sometimes located inside the vaginal opening.

U-SPOT: This doughnut-shaped area surrounding the urethra fills with blood and becomes sensitive when you're sexually aroused. (In fact, touching it is only pleasurable with proper arousal and plenty of lubrication!) And you'll probably find it doesn't need much pressure. The U-spot is the beginning of the famed G-spot, which extends internally along the front wall of the vagina.

CLITORIS

The **CLITORAL HEAD**, or **GLANS**, is often very sensitive, even too sensitive—especially when you're touching it before you are aroused. It has more than 8,000 nerve endings: more than any other part of the human body! Because it's hidden under the clitoral hood, it might be difficult to see.

Extending from the clitoral head, the **CLITORAL SHAFT** ducks up and underneath the hood. Like the shaft of the penis, it's not usually as sensitive as the head, but stimulating it through the clitoral hood still offers a lot of sensation.

The **CLITORAL LEGS** look like the two longer parts of a turkey's wishbone. Because they're located deeper inside the body, they're a bit harder to stimulate. Moving a toy, penis, or finger in a side-to-side motion while inserted shallowly into the vagina may stimulate the clitoral legs.

The **VESTIBULAR BULBS** are located beneath the skin's surface, between the inner and outer labia, and attach to the shaft of the clitoris. Increased blood flow to the area during sexual arousal causes this erectile tissue to puff up and change color.

BELOW THE SURFACE

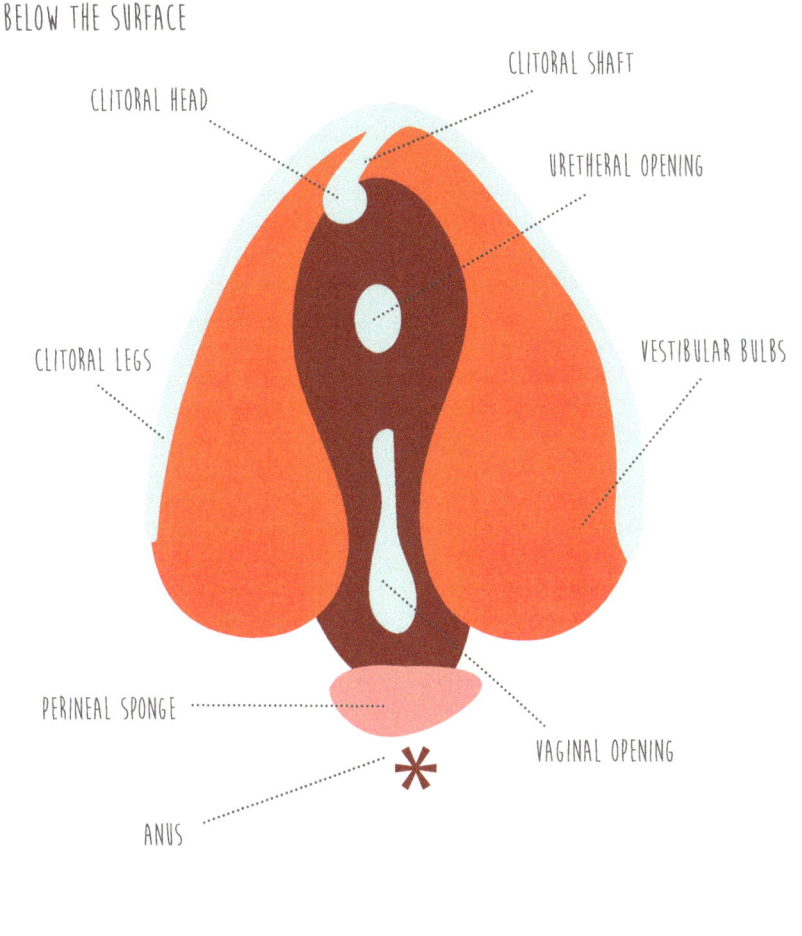

CLITORAL HEAD

CLITORAL SHAFT

URETHERAL OPENING

CLITORAL LEGS

VESTIBULAR BULBS

PERINEAL SPONGE

VAGINAL OPENING

ANUS

SIMILAR BUT DIFFERENT

In utero, differentiation of the sexual organs happens at around seven weeks. Although they look quite different to one another, the tissues in male and female bodies are similar. The head of the clitoris is homologous, or similar to, the head of the penis: it's the same thing in a smaller package. The outer labia are homologous to the scrotum; the clitoral hood is similar to the foreskin; and the vestibular bulbs are equivalent to the bulb or base of the penis, which is located behind the testicles.

SOME PEOPLE ARE INTERSEX

Some people are born with a mix of **XX** (female) and **XY** (male) chromosomes, which means they're a combination of both sexes. The genitals of some intersex people look different from birth, while others have less physical differentiation and don't discover that they're intersex until they're older—for example, when trying to conceive a child. Because all bodies grow out of the same tissue, some of these erogenous zones may look a little different or be located in slightly different spots on an intersex person. Some intersex people may have had surgeries as babies—a practice that's generally being discouraged these days—and that can alter the location of some pleasure centers. But they're still there—and they're definitely worth looking for!

PERINEUM: This is the sensitive tissue located between the vagina and the anus. Generally, it likes either a super-light touch or firm pressure, and not much in between. This area can be torn during childbirth, and any subsequent scarring can make it feel less sensitive.

ANUS: The anus has as many nerve endings as we have in our fingertips. (Enough said!) Even just external anal play can feel absolutely divine.

INSIDE THE VAGINA

OPENING: The opening to the vagina has lots of nerve endings (and that means it can be a major source of pleasure!), but we often don't pay enough attention to this area because of what we've been told constitutes "great" (that is, penis-centric) intercourse: bigger, harder, deeper. Tune in to this sensitive area: Touching and stroking it shallowly can feel fantastic.

PERINEAL SPONGE: This is erectile tissue that's located between the anus and the vagina, about a thumb's depth inside the vagina and toward its back wall. You can feel it by placing one finger inside the vagina and/or one inside the anus. Stimulating the perineal sponge and the perineum at the same time can be incredibly pleasurable.

URETHRAL SPONGE OR G-SPOT: The G-spot isn't really a spot at all: It's more of a G-stretch, or a piece of tissue about 1 to 3 inches (2.5 to 7.5 cm) long that's located on the front wall of the vagina, anywhere from a knuckle's depth to a full finger's depth inside. That said, the G-spot is not situated *in* the vagina: because it's erectile tissue that surrounds the urethra, you feel it *through* the front wall of the vagina. On some women it bulges into that front wall, while other women require pressure in order to feel it through the vaginal wall.

A-SPOT, OR ANTERIOR FORNIX EROGENOUS ZONE (AFE): Also known as the "second G-spot," this sensitive area is also located on the front wall of the vagina, but it's deeper inside than the G-spot, and isn't as spongy or rippled. It might be harder to reach using your fingers alone.

CERVIX: The cervix is the entrance to the uterus, and it's about ¾ to 1 ¼ inches (2 to 3 cm) long, with a very small opening that's just big enough to allow fluid (like semen and menstrual blood) to move in and out. It's an erogenous zone for some women, especially when it's

bumped gently by a toy, fingers, or a penis, but it can be very uncomfortable for others, so explore carefully.

CUL-DE-SAC: When the vagina elongates with arousal to accommodate penetration, it leaves a little pouch, or cul-de-sac, behind the cervix. It's one of the lesser-known erogenous zones because it's a bit harder to reach, but stimulating it can be intensely pleasurable. Accessing the cul-de-sac usually requires deeper thrusting, or the insertion of small metal "ben wa" balls deep into the vagina before penetration.

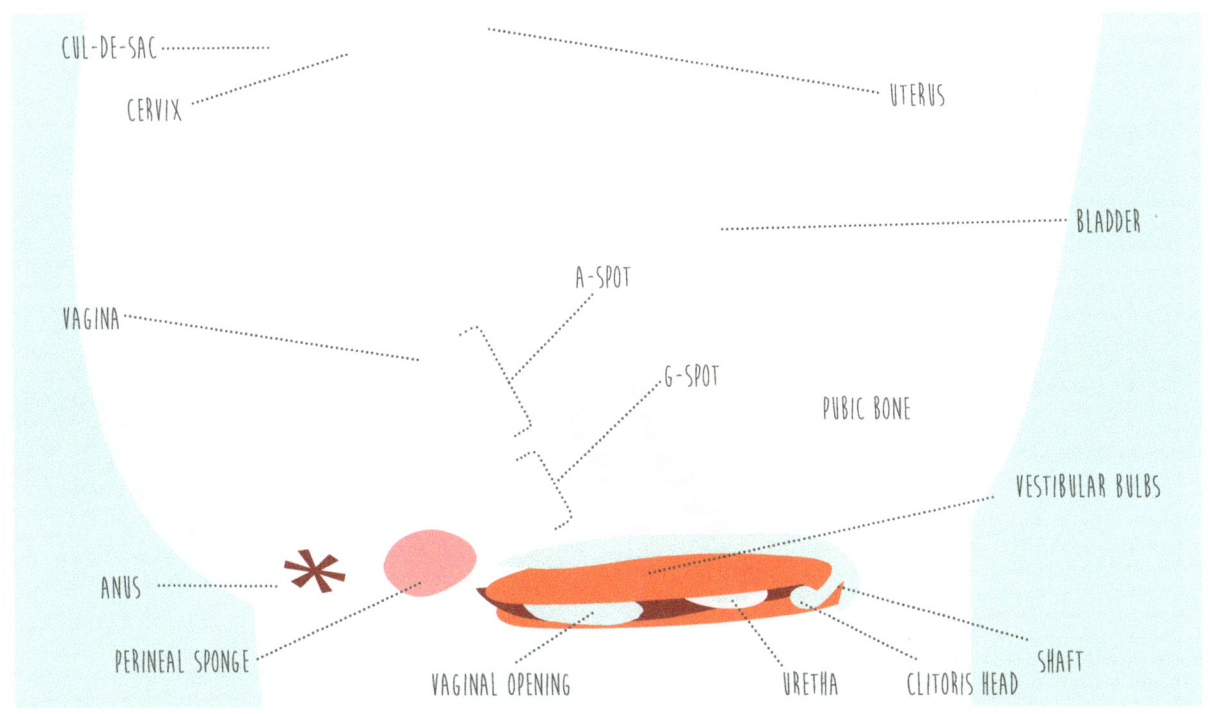

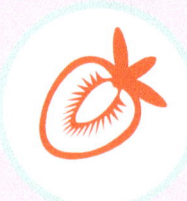

FOUR WAYS TO FIND YOUR G-SPOT

Haven't found your G-spot yet? Here are a few ways to help you get there:

—— 1 ——

MAKE SURE YOU'RE REALLY, REALLY AROUSED. To be able to feel your G-spot with your fingers—and to make it feel good—you have to get plenty of blood flowing to the area. (It'll feel rippled and spongy, like a balloon filled with a little bit of water.) And that means you need to be in the mood. Wait to go exploring until you're relaxed, aroused, and lubricated.

—— 2 ——

GO SHALLOW. For some women, the G-spot is located 2 to 3 inches (5 to 7.5 cm) inside the vagina, while for others, it's barely one knuckle deep. Gravity may have something to do with it; unless you do plenty of Kegel exercises, age and pregnancy can cause your pelvic floor to slip downward, and these erogenous zones may shift closer to the vaginal opening. So be sure to pay attention to what you feel when you touch and stroke the first inch (2.5 cm) of your vagina.

—— 3 ——

USE PLENTY OF PRESSURE. Because the G-spot is composed of erectile tissue that surrounds the urethra, it can only be stimulated through the vaginal wall. Some women respond to very little pressure, while others need more substantial pressure from very firm fingers or toys, such as those made of steel, glass, or firm silicone.

—— 4 ——

PULL, DON'T PUSH. We often think of intercourse as an inward thrust, but a "pulling out" motion can stimulate your G-spot more effectively. Slide your (or your partner's) fingers inside you, and then make a "come hither" motion with your fingers as you pull them out. If you're using a toy instead, use one with a bulbous head for better effect; angle it toward your belly button and then pull it out toward the opening of the vagina. Or, if you're having intercourse with a partner, get your partner to do the same thing with his penis or a strap-on dildo, angling it toward your belly button and then pulling it out. If your partner has a penis, this motion also pulls against the coronal ridge at the base of the head, and he'll love the sensation.

BODY CHANGES

Change is a natural part of life. Thanks to things like hormonal shifts, childbirth, medications, lifestyle habits, and plain old gravity, your body will look and feel different as you age. Here's a rundown of what to expect at the milestones in your sexual lifecycle.

PUBERTY

Hair grows on your vulva, armpits, and nipples. Your breasts begin to grow, and your hips, butt, vulva, thighs, and upper arms develop more fatty tissue. Vaginal walls thicken, and your vagina starts to produce a pale or colorless discharge. That discharge is completely normal, by the way; it's simply the body's way of cleaning itself.

WHAT'S THAT WHITE STUFF IN MY UNDERWEAR?

Aside from the natural discharge the vagina produces, the cervix also produces a discharge, typically twice a month. As the gateway between the uterus and the vagina, the cervix performs an important function: it allows sperm in while keeping the uterus clean, safe, and ready for a baby (if there is one). It produces different types of mucus depending on where you are in your menstrual cycle. Unless you're pregnant, just before your period (day 1), your cervix gets rid of the protective plug that guarded the uterus. Because you're not having a baby, the cervix can now let out the accumulated blood. Just before ovulation (around day 14, when an egg is pulled into the fallopian tube), it unplugs itself again, producing a different substance that makes it easy for sperm to pass through. (Our bodies also produce different types of discharge at other stages of the menstrual cycle.)

These forms of discharge are perfectly natural and healthy. For more information on how to track your cycle (including a handy app!), check out the Justisse Method (www. justisse.ca).

PREGNANCY

During pregnancy, hormones and increased blood flow dramatically change the vagina and vulva, and you might notice that your vaginal area is especially moist or "wet." Unless your medical practitioner advises you against sex and orgasm, you don't need to stop enjoying sexual pleasure when you're pregnant. Although everyone is different, many women find that nausea and fatigue in the first trimester make sex much less appealing. Luckily, that doesn't last forever: the second trimester is often the "randy" phase, when nausea diminishes, energy returns, and sex starts to sound good again. By the third trimester, you might start to feel uncomfortable as your due date approaches, so it's likely that sex will be less gymnastic. (Some women also report that orgasms are more difficult to achieve and are less intense.) But no two women's experiences are exactly the same, so comfort levels and responses to sexual pleasure will vary from woman to woman, and from pregnancy to pregnancy. Always follow the golden rule of what feels good to you!

HOW DO I CLEAN MY VAGINA?

Relax: there's no need to clean your machine. The human body is very good at self-regulating, so you don't have to put anything at all inside your vagina to clean it. Our bodies are home to ten thousand different types of helpful bacteria, and some live inside the vagina. These "good" bacteria help keep your vaginal ecosystem balanced. Messing with the system—by douching, for example—can actually throw off your vagina's bacterial balance. That's because douching gets rid of all the bacteria, and it's typically the unwanted or "bad" bacteria that come back first and make your vagina their home. If you notice a very strong odor or an unusual discharge, see your doctor to make sure you don't have an infection, because some infections can lead to infertility or other problems. Also, see your doctor if you think you might have a yeast infection. They're pretty common, and they're usually accompanied by itching, burning, and thicker vaginal discharge. They can be treated with natural remedies or prescription drugs.

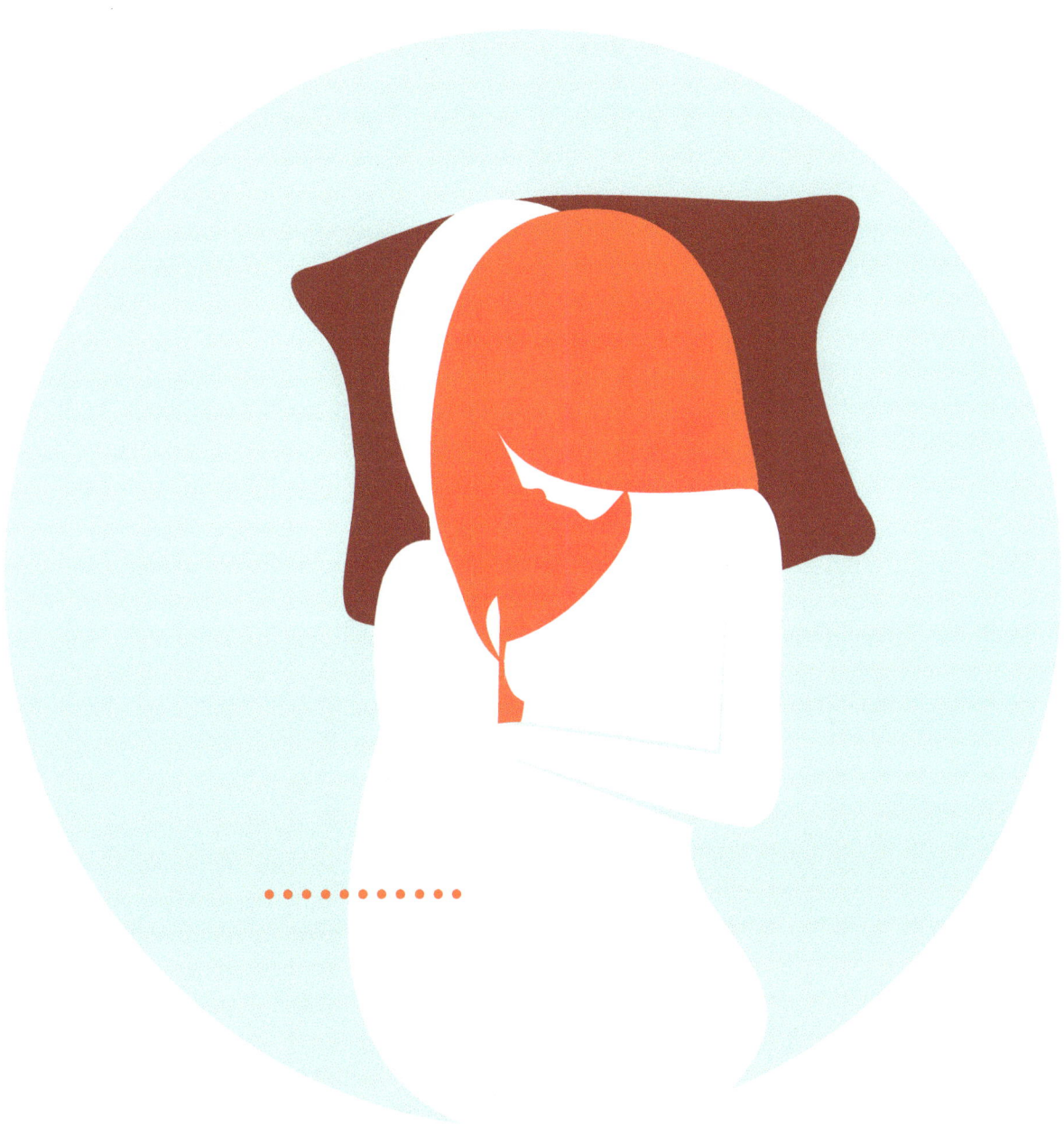

POST-PREGNANCY

When it comes to post-pregnancy sex, doctors often advise holding off for about six weeks, so that your perineum has time to heal and your cervix can fully close before you try vaginal penetration again. But that rule is pretty flexible: Some women enjoy vaginal stimulation within hours of childbirth, while others prefer to wait longer than six weeks before giving sex a go. Either way, external play can be lots of fun during this time—either instead of or in conjunction with penetrative sex. (And that goes for both partner and solo sex.) Whichever way you like to play, though, if you're breast-feeding, you'll probably have to keep a bottle of lube nearby during sex. Your new temporary hormonal balance dries you up, trying to discourage you from making another baby because your body is already occupied in caring for one (or more!) and would prefer to wait a while before embarking on the stressful job of producing another one. It's also possible that you won't enjoy breast stimulation while breast-feeding. Some women do, which is perfectly healthy, but others might feel conflicted: Are breasts wonderful sources of sexual pleasure, or are they functional organs that are there to sustain a baby? Of course, the two aren't mutually exclusive, but trying to combine them makes some women feel uncomfortable. And, of course, it's possible that you'll be downright sick of having your breasts groped and mauled all day by the baby, and the less attention they get, the better, thank you very much!

MENOPAUSE

The decrease in estrogen that accompanies menopause changes our bodies—especially our sexual organs. You'll probably notice that your periods will become less regular, and your menstrual flow will be less predictable: Sometimes you'll lose less blood, sometimes more. Your breasts may feel sore, and your vaginal walls may start to thin out or even atrophy. In terms of sexual pleasure, this means you might not find breast or vaginal stimulation as pleasurable as you used to. Having orgasms might become more challenging, too.

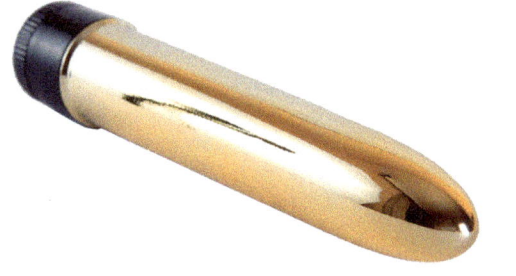

These changes don't mean you have to have to say goodbye to sexual pleasure for good. Here are a few ways to keep solo or partner sex comfortable—and exciting—during menopause:

1. LUBRICANT, LUBRICANT, LUBRICANT. Lube makes fingers, toys, and penises glide more smoothly during sex internally and externally, and it minimizes any discomfort during penetration. (Check out page 67 to find out which type of lubricant is right for you.)

2. USE IT OR LOSE IT. Plenty of blood flow to your erogenous zones keeps thinning vaginal walls healthy and strong. And the best way to keep the blood flowing? Sex! Whether it's on your own or with a partner, regular stimulation of the genital area helps keep it healthy and receptive to pleasure.

3. TRY A VIBRATOR. Leading gynecologist Dr. Mary Jane Minkin recommends that women in menopause use vibrators regularly to maintain their sexual health. They have other benefits, too: if you need a little more intensity to reach orgasm than you used to, or if you just want to switch things up a bit, a vibrator can be a fabulous addition to sex play. (Chapter 5 will help you choose one.)

4. FOCUS ON WHAT FEELS GOOD. Follow your bliss, as the saying goes, and do more of what feels pleasurable. If you don't enjoy vaginal penetration, don't do it! Stimulating your vulva, clitoris, or inner labia will still increase blood flow to your genitals by making you feel aroused, and that's what benefits your vaginal walls. Remember that sex can be a full-body experience, so enjoy rediscovering your new body as it changes.

Your body is your own, and it's yours to enjoy throughout your sexual life span. Now it's time to get down to business! Chapter 3 will show you how to get started when it comes to self-pleasure— and you might just find that you're the best lover you've ever had.

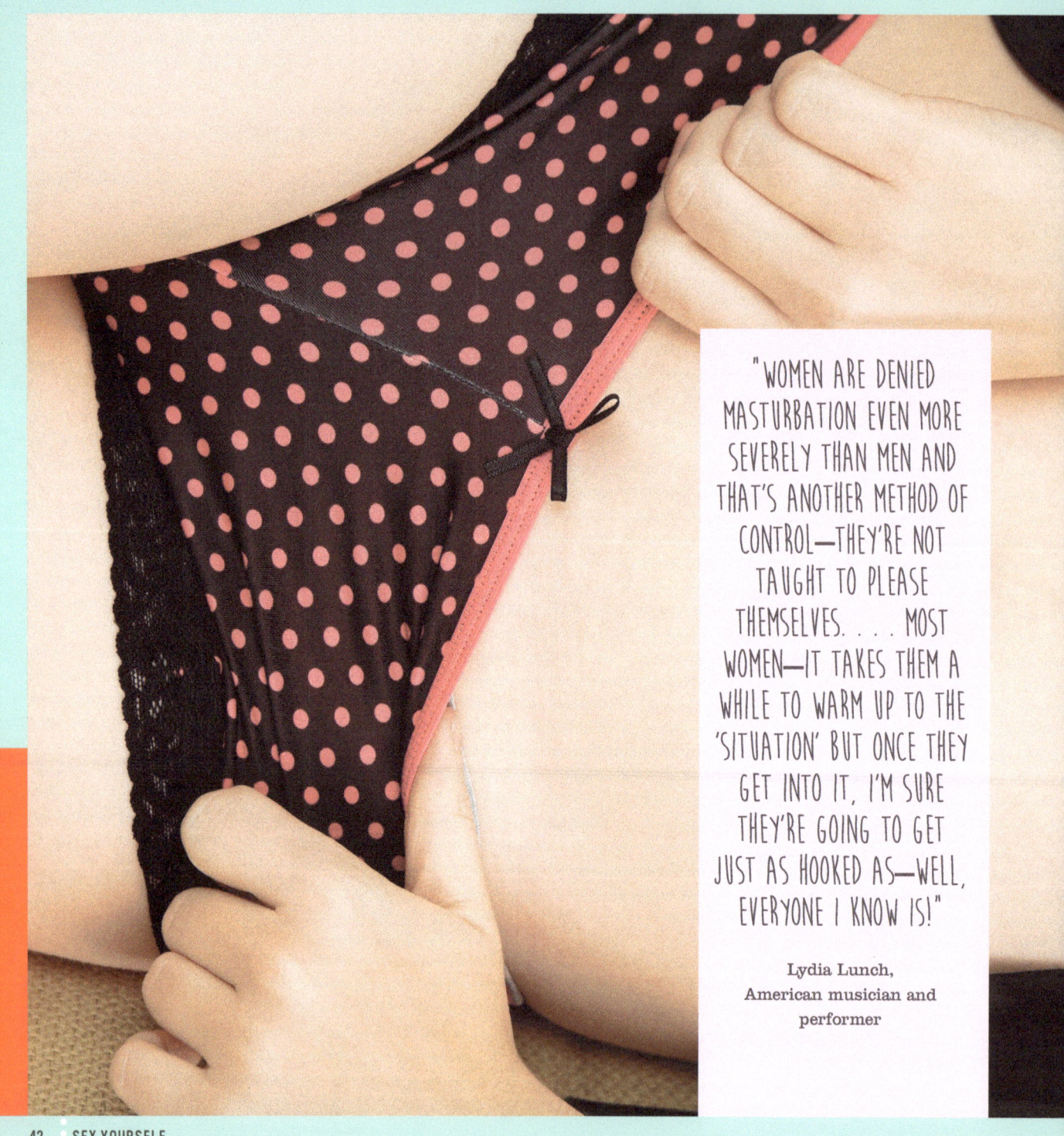

"WOMEN ARE DENIED MASTURBATION EVEN MORE SEVERELY THAN MEN AND THAT'S ANOTHER METHOD OF CONTROL—THEY'RE NOT TAUGHT TO PLEASE THEMSELVES. . . . MOST WOMEN—IT TAKES THEM A WHILE TO WARM UP TO THE 'SITUATION' BUT ONCE THEY GET INTO IT, I'M SURE THEY'RE GOING TO GET JUST AS HOOKED AS—WELL, EVERYONE I KNOW IS!"

Lydia Lunch,
American musician and
performer

3

KICK-STARTING
PLEASURE:
DISCOVERING YOUR EROTIC POTENTIAL

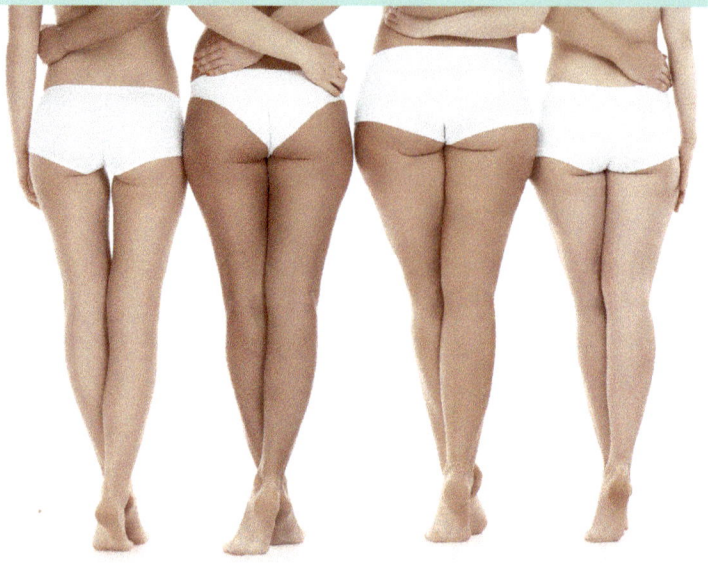

● ● ● ● ● ● ● ● ● ● ●

Who hasn't been for a spin on the relationship merry-go-round? Crushes, lust, passion, flings, committed relationships, breakups, we've all been there. Partners may come and go, but there's one relationship you have that isn't going anywhere: your relationship with you. Your body, emotions, and desires are your own, and they'll always be a part of you, no matter what. After all, it's impossible to break up with yourself! So honor that relationship: Make friends with yourself and start loving your body right now, because the truth is—whether you've got a partner or not—you're dating yourself.

It's easy to let other people define our sexuality for us, or to allow it to revolve around someone else. (Women are particularly susceptible to that tendency.) But the fact is, the way in which you respond to your own sexuality is unique: it arises from and expresses itself via internal and external cues that are specific to you. And that means it's yours alone. Sure, you might express your sexual self differently when your crush is in the room, or if you're out at a nightclub with friends, or when you're interacting online or on social media sites. Your various and shifting responses to those environments and cues are part of your sexual self, which is a vital part of who you are. And it's

just as important to stay tuned in to it as it is to stay connected to your emotional, physical, and spiritual selves. When you take back—and take charge of—your sexual power, you can choose the ways in which you cultivate, express, and act upon your sexuality.

This chapter will help you do just that. In the coming pages, you'll learn how to enhance your erotic potential; you'll explore pleasure zones and arousal options; and you'll learn to give yourself permission to feel good, which is the key to enjoying self-pleasure. Remember that sex, solo or partnered, doesn't have to revolve around the penis-in-vagina model. Instead, it's about what feels good to you in the present moment, depending upon your specific desires; the mood you're in; how much energy you have; and the itch you want to scratch, so to speak. And because solo sex can only enhance sex with your partner, boosting your sexual self-esteem and exercising your libido will only make partner sex even better. (Or, if you're looking to attract a partner, know that your increased confidence and newly awakened passions will help you do just that!)

LOVE YOUR BODY

We've heard it a million times, but it's so true: having great sex means loving your body first. And that's not always easy. Lots of us struggle with our self-image—and the media's narrow representations of "sexy" certainly don't help, because they value a single type of beauty that very few people can achieve or maintain. In addition, popular images of women usually feature traditional markers of femininity, like long hair, skirts, and high heels—excluding the alternative, equally valid options of other gender expressions, such as androgynous, genderqueer, or butch. To make matters even worse, we receive very clear messages about who "deserves" sexual pleasure: those who conform to this traditional model of beauty are "worthy" of it because of their physical characteristics, while those who don't, aren't. And it's difficult to embrace pleasure—from yourself or anyone else—and to enjoy feeling sexy if you don't feel worthy of it in the first place.

Let's trash this boring, confining definition of beauty! The truth is that all of us deserve pleasure and "sexy" is completely subjective; it comes in all shapes, sizes, colors, and ages. So many of us are awfully self-critical when it comes to appearance, and we stress about every single curve or blemish. That's exhausting, isn't it? It's time to give yourself a break, and to stop letting pop culture define what's sexy and what isn't. Find more diverse role models to inspire you instead, and surround yourself with images of people who are confident in their wrinkles, bulges, sags, scars, and stretch marks. It's not hard to find them: there are plenty of resources online and in print reclaiming these bodies as beautiful and sexy. (Check out the Resources section on page 168.) Just like laughter, sexiness is infectious: When you start to embrace yours, other people will appreciate and admire it, too. (Really!)

Of course, we all feel insecure about some aspects of our physical selves. That's perfectly normal, but you don't have to let those insecurities trample your sex life. Changing your attitude toward parts of your physical self, such as your age, fertility, ability level, or the presence of pain or illness, can help you get in touch with your sexual self. Here are a few ways to start.

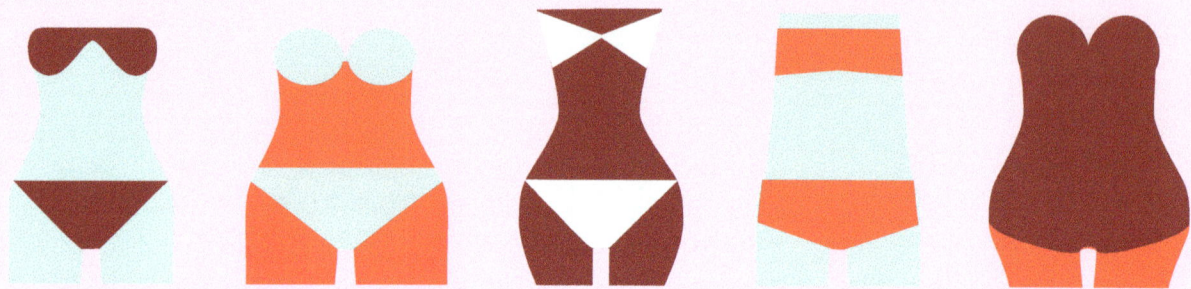

"THE FIRST TIME I MASTURBATED WAS AFTER I HAD SEX A FEW TIMES WITH MY 'FIRST' AT AGE 23. I WAS SO FRUSTRATED THAT HE KNEW MY BODY BETTER THAN I DID. AS A WOMAN WITH A NEUROLOGICAL DISABILITY, I HAD NEVER BEEN ABLE TO TOUCH MYSELF BEFORE, BUT AS THE URGE GREW, SO TOO DID MY YEARNING TO FIND A WAY. IT REQUIRED ASSISTANCE TO GET INTO THE RIGHT POSITION. IT ISN'T EASY FOR OTHERS TO UNDERSTAND, AS MOST PEOPLE SEE PEOPLE LIKE ME AS ASEXUAL. SOMETIMES I SIT IN MY CHAIR, FULLY CLOTHED, ROCKING BACK AND FORTH, WATCHING PORN ON XHAMSTER.COM UNTIL I'M FINALLY ABLE TO ORGASM, BREATHLESS AND CONTENT."

Stella Darkely
www.scandalouswheeliegirl.com

• • • • • • • • • • •

LOVE YOUR AGE

Western society's obsession with youth tries to convince us that younger is, by definition, sexier. Sure, all puppies are cute, but it's impossible to reduce sexiness to something as simple as a number. Sexual attractiveness is far more nuanced than that, and it doesn't depend on your ability to twist yourself into gymnastic sex positions. Plus, age offers some serious advantages. The older you are, the more sex you've had, and you're more likely to be open to new sexual experiences than you were when you were younger. There's no replacement for the wisdom that comes with a few years of living: you've had way more sex than when you were younger, and that's incredibly exciting! And solo play is an optimal way to discover even more sources of pleasure.

UNDERSTAND YOUR FERTILITY

Fertility issues can affect our attitudes toward our femininity and, therefore, our sexuality. Infertility can be a result of genetics, age, illness, or surgery, among other factors, but no matter what causes it, having trouble conceiving or being diagnosed as infertile can be shocking, stressful, and painful. It can even make many women wonder whether they're relationship-worthy at all. If you're struggling with fertility issues, consider working through them with a therapist or counselor, and let your friends, family, and partner support you. And remember that being unable to conceive doesn't make you any less sexy. Conception is just one reason for having sex: You can still enjoy sex for its physical pleasure, the emotional connection it offers, and its health benefits. There's no doubt that it's important to mourn the loss of this part of you, but don't let it erase your whole erotic being and expression.

MANAGE PAIN AND ABILITY LEVELS

Although the media is beginning to represent differently "abled" role models—that is, people with different levels of physical ability—it still shies away from depicting people with physical disabilities as sexual beings. This stereotype is slowly changing, but you can create your own role models, too. People with disabilities can, should, and do have healthy, satisfying, happy sex lives—and that includes you. If your body has changed as a result of a disability or from having to manage pain, it may take time for you to adjust to your new limits and preferences. What's more, you might be angry with your body and its new limitations: You might wish you could still do things the way you used to, or in the way it seems that "everyone else" can. That's perfectly understandable. Remember, though, that everyone's bodies and sexual preferences are different, regardless of ability level.

You might be able to experience pleasure and enjoy sex in different ways than you used to, or you might prefer other types of sex than the vaginal intercourse-focused expressions of sexuality that tend to be so dominant. Enter solo sex! There's no better way to explore new desires and preferences, so take some time to appreciate your own body, and to figure out which sensations and positions work for you. Take note of the times of day when you feel at your best, or when side effects of medication are at a minimum, and think about enjoying solo sex during these times.

Lastly, don't be afraid to talk about your new sex life with those in the know, like your doctor, a sex educator, or local support groups; chances are, you'll learn new ways to make sex—solo or partnered—even better.

HANDLE AN STI DIAGNOSIS

Sexually transmitted infections (STIs) are surprisingly common. About 65 to 90 percent of sexually active people have herpes—most of them undiagnosed—and most sexually active people will have contracted HPV at some point before the age of thirty. (Luckily, your body fights off 90 percent of HPV infections naturally, in the same way that it combats the viruses that cause the common cold.) But even though STIs are so common, the experience of having one unfortunately still carries a lot of stigma, and it can make many people uncomfortable with enjoying sexual pleasure—especially with a partner. Being diagnosed with an STI doesn't mean deep-sixing your sex life, though. It's true that negotiating safer sex with a new partner can be a delicate conversation, but it's perfectly doable,

and you can create hot safer sex with someone else. And what's more, sex with yourself is perfectly safe and fabulously satisfying—no awkward discussion required! (Just be sure to use condoms on toys if you're switching from anal to vaginal play.) So don't say goodbye to great sex: Get comfortable with negotiating partner sex in new ways, and get busy enjoying your own body.

EMBRACE YOUR POST-SURGERY SELF

If you've had surgery as a result of illness—especially breast, gynecological, or anal illnesses—accepting your altered body as "new and improved" can be challenging. The beauty norms perpetuated by popular media might not represent your body these days. But that doesn't mean you're any less sexy than you were before your illness. If feeling sexy is a struggle at first, that's okay, it's not just you. Check out support groups in your area, or strike up informal discussions with other survivors, and get excited about re-envisioning what beauty means to you. Implants, tattoos, or new or different clothes and accessories are options that might help you rediscover your own personal sexy. Always remember that you're not alone, and that if other people have forged ahead with full sex lives post-illness, you can, too.

CELEBRATE THE POSITIVE (AND THERE ARE LOTS OF POSITIVES!)

Don't be a hater. Instead of focusing on what you don't like about your body, remind yourself of all the ways that you are hot, sexy, and attractive. Whether you've got big or small breasts, large or small labia, a thick, curvy body or a skinny, angular one, every part of your body is beautiful in its own way. And the grass isn't always greener: Each feature has its advantages and disadvantages. For example, large breasts can really fill out an outfit—but small breasts don't cause back problems. Larger bodies offer lush, enticing curves, while lightweight frames make acrobatic sex easier. Large labia are pleasurable to play with during solo or partner sex, but small labia are less likely to get in the way of penetration, and can make stimulating other erogenous zones, such as the clitoris, that much easier. The moral of the story is, your body's unique features can give you pleasure in immeasurable ways. (And whatever you do, don't compare yourself to others. It's a destructive practice that'll rarely leave you feeling good about yourself. The fact is that no one will ever have the same awesome mix of characteristics that you do. So focus on the infinite beauties of your own body; a little exploratory solo sex is a great way to start.)

BOOST YOUR LIBIDO—AND DO IT TODAY

The best way to put yourself in the mood for solo (or partnered) sex is to make sexiness a part of your life—every day. Why? Well, it's tough to suddenly snap into feeling and acting sexual if you don't make it a regular habit. By the same token, tuning in to your erotic self is smooth sailing when sexy is your default setting. That's why it's so important to discover what makes you feel hot, confident, and strong. Here are a few easy ways to do just that.

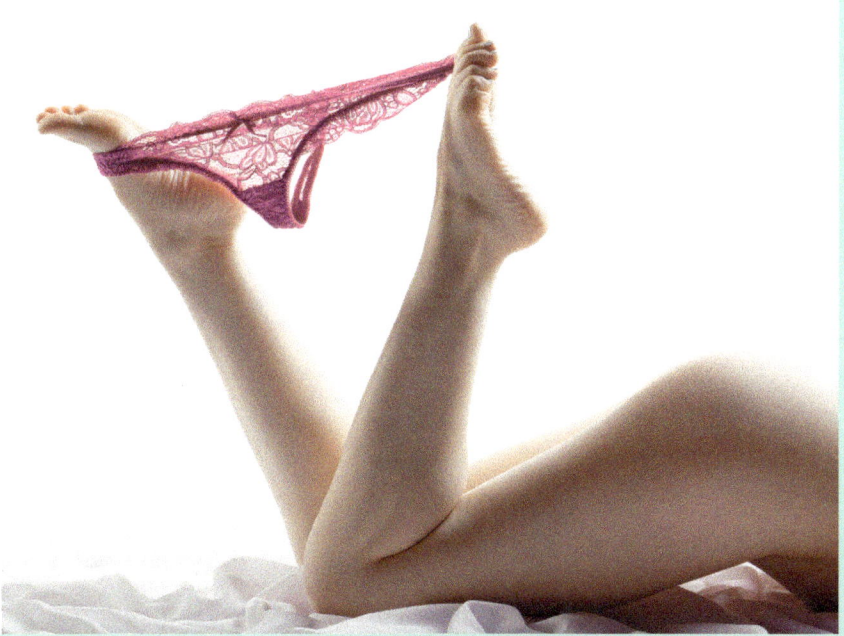

DRESS UP

Just for today, put away the sweatpants, the baggy T-shirts, and those seven-year-old jeans you can't bear to part with. Sexy clothes don't require a special occasion—so go ahead and slip into your best lingerie, your sexiest dress, or your favorite leatherwear, whether or not you've got a hot date with a partner or yourself. Choose an outfit that makes you feel attractive and assertive. Wear lingerie that makes you feel strong under your street clothes. You'll notice that you're suddenly standing up straight, speaking up for yourself, smiling a lot, and enjoying your own body—and others will start to notice that, too.

FLIRT

Once you've donned your sexy attire, notice people whom you find attractive. When you see someone who flips your pancake, smile or make eye contact with her or him. In the morning, give yourself a little more time to saunter, rather than race, to work. Let your hips sway a little more than usual, and pay attention to how good it feels to move in your own body. Even if you're shy, flirt gently in a way that's authentic to you. (As long as you're respectful, it's fine to use a little sensual undertone to engage people.) Then run over these experiences in your mind; they'll make great fantasy material for your solo-pleasure session later on!

CONNECT

Once or twice a day, take a risk and offer someone a respectful compliment. Telling your coworker you want to jump his or her bones doesn't count as respectful, but it's fine to tell a person that she looks great, that his ideas in the meeting gave you some food for thought, or that her professionalism is inspiring. These are all positive ways to reach out and connect with others. Giving genuine compliments is one of life's great pleasures, and it can boost your own confidence, too. And, as we know, more confidence means better sex!

BE A PLEASURE SEEKER

Sex isn't just about what's between your legs, so be sure to seize the pleasure that's part of everyday activities. For example, the act of eating is a physical necessity, but it can also be a sensuous experience. Pay attention to food's texture and the way flavors meld into one another. Eat with your hands when possible. Make some "ohh" sounds out loud as you slowly savor your favorite treat. When you're walking down the street, put down your phone so that you really notice the world around you. See if you can decipher the different smells in the air as you walk through the neighborhood. At home, play some music and really listen to it, instead of multitasking and making dinner at the same time. Take in the wild sounds of children playing in the playground. When you're dressing and undressing, do it slowly and relish the sensation of the fabric against your skin. Look at yourself in the mirror while you're doing it or pretend that you're putting on a show for someone else. Read erotic books that'll take you to places that feel sexy and exciting: Novels are great for full character development and deliciously drawn-out anticipation, while short stories can supply you with fantasies and ideas to add to your erotic repertoire. That way, when you're ready to get it on—well, you won't have far to go.

EXERCISE AT YOUR OWN PACE

You don't have to run a marathon to reap the benefits of exercise. A little moderate movement will get your blood pumping, boost your energy, improve your self-confidence, and jump-start your libido. If you're not much of an athlete, start with walking a little during your commute. Get off the bus a stop or two earlier than usual and walk the rest of the way, or go for a stroll on your lunch break. Or try dancing; moving your body in graceful, sexy ways can help

make sensual expression feel more natural to you. Any form of dance you enjoy will do the trick, so sign up for a class, or just turn up the tunes and groove in your own living room. Try to exercise regularly even when you're not in the mood: it replenishes energy—and that includes sexual energy.

EAT THE GOOD STUFF

Consuming healthy, unprocessed foods and eating between five and nine portions of fruits and vegetables daily is essential for good health, but some of these natural foods have another handy side benefit. Avocados, almonds, arugula, seafood (especially oysters), figs, and

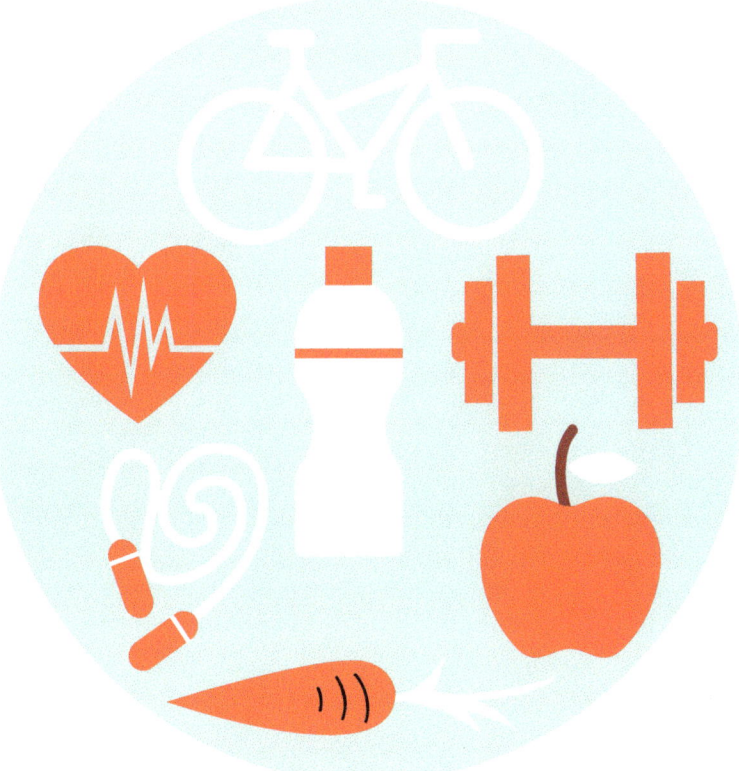

citrus fruits are all said to be aphrodisiacs! So are supplements such as yohimbe, damiana, gingko, ginseng, horny goat weed, wild yam, and maca root, which are available in health food stores. Don't expect these aphrodisiacs to magically transform you into a sex machine, though: their effects are usually pretty subtle, and may affect some people more strongly than others. (And always consult your doctor before you try them.)

ADJUST YOUR EXPECTATIONS

When it comes to arousal, women are generally a little slower to boil than men are. So don't expect your arousal to zoom from zero to sixty in an unreasonable amount of time. Those of us with lower libidos are like slow cookers: We need small, consistent doses of arousal to keep our fires burning. That's why keeping pleasure on your radar is such a good idea: it means you won't need to put in as much effort to turn up the heat when you're ready to get it on. If your pot is already simmering, you'll just need a little boost to bring it to a rollicking boil!

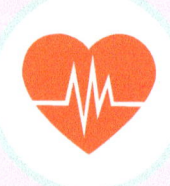

KEEP YOUR LIBIDO IN SHAPE

Okay, so you're down with making sexiness part of yourself on a day-to-day basis. But what do you do when life gets in the way? Your sexual self is just one part of the complex, multifaceted person you are, and it's intimately connected to your physical and emotional self. Here's how to keep pleasure on the menu when:

....

PARENTHOOD FEELS OVERWHELMING. Maybe you're coming to grips with breast-feeding; you've got a newborn, and haven't slept a wink in weeks; you feel drained by your intense emotional connection to your kids; you're chauffeuring the kids from one activity to another; or you're stressed out from trying to conceive.

WHY NOT: Ask for help, or hire a sitter? While these concerns are definitely pressing, you can still take time out. Carve out some time to connect with yourself or your partner. Make yourself and your relationship a priority; your kids will benefit in the long-term by seeing you, their role model, care for herself. If you're single, think about dating, go dancing with friends, or do whatever else helps you nurture your sexual self. Don't forget solo activities like luxurious baths, erotic books or films, or dressing up. Making yourself feel good doesn't mean ignoring the kids, it means taking as little as five minutes daily to recharge and reawaken your sexual self.

....

EMOTIONALLY, YOU'RE FEELING FRAGILE. It's possible that your relationship isn't as strong as you'd like it to be. Perhaps you're not feeling as connected to your partner as you'd like, or you're struggling with unresolved issues, like a loss of control or power, or you're not feeling positive about yourself and your place in life.

WHY NOT: Talk to caring friends, and/or a therapist? Sharing your challenges raises your self-esteem, and helps you make empowering choices. Be direct with your partner, and seek help from a counselor together so that you can work through conflicts and express your desires to one another. Come up with a specific, realistic plan to help you move towards your emotional, physical, spiritual, intimate, and professional goals.

PERSONAL ISSUES ARISE. Staying interested in sex is a tall order if you're grappling with a fear of intimacy, low physical or sexual self-esteem, the aftereffects or trauma or abuse, or an unsatisfying sexual relationship.

WHY NOT: Start with a book? A workbook like *Healing Sex: A Mind-Body Approach to Healing Sexual Trauma* by Staci Haines can help you begin to address painful issues like these. When you're ready, talking to a trusted friend or therapist can also be useful. If you're unsure about your sex skills, why not brush up on them a bit? Whether it's oral sex, hand jobs, stripping, or just flirting, books, DVDs, and workshops in your area can help you explore what both you and a partner might like.

LIFESTYLE HABITS GET YOU DOWN. It's so easy to let bad habits slide for a little too long. If you've found yourself overly stressed, in a sedentary lifestyle, consuming too much alcohol, or relying on a diet that's high in processed foods, sugar, or fat, chances are that sex won't be as much of a priority.

WHY NOT: Cut back on processed stuff—and the alcohol, too? You don't need it to relax. Instead, do a little exercise every day. Turn off the computer and TV, and get involved in a project or hobby that you love. Meditate daily. Or try doing just one activity a day—such as cooking and eating—slowly, purposefully, and mindfully.

PHYSICAL CONDITIONS NEED ATTENTION. If you're suffering from depression, anxiety, heart disease, sleep disorders, menopause, STIs, or genital pain, you need to seek relief for these conditions before you can focus on your sex life.

WHY NOT: Follow your medical professional's advice on dealing with your medical challenges while seeking a second opinion as well? Lots of people find alternative therapies, such as traditional Chinese medicine or naturopathy, very helpful. If painful sex is a problem, read *When Sex Hurts: A Woman's Guide to Banishing Sexual Pain* by Andrew Goldstein. It's a fabulous resource that can help you nail down the specifics of genital pain. Pay attention to the time of day when you're at your best and most alert, or when the side effects of medications or your condition will be at a minimum, and consider enjoying a little solo or partnered pleasure during these times. Experiment with pleasure even if you don't feel sexy at first; often the very act of trying boosts our mood and helps us feel sexier.

MEDICATIONS AFFECT YOUR MOOD AND LIBIDO. Antidepressants (SSRIs), antihistamines, steroids, anticholinergics, medications that treat incontinence, anti-hypertensives, and the birth control pill can all make a difference in your sex drive.

WHY NOT: Try different brands of the same medication? Some antidepressants, like Wellbutrin, tend to have fewer negative sexual side effects than other SSRIs. Ask your health care professional if there are other medications or natural options that might minimize the side effects. Visit a sexual health clinic, such as Planned Parenthood, to determine whether a different form of birth control might work better for you.

EASING INTO SELF-PLEASURE

You've taken time to get to know your sexual self, and you love the idea of solo sex. But what if, when theory meets practice, the idea of pleasuring yourself still feels ... weird? That's completely understandable. Although both men and women receive mixed messages about masturbation and partner sex from our parents, peers, and society at large, women are more likely to be discouraged from masturbating than men are. That's because women have been taught that being "good"—that is, worthy of a partner's affection—means being sexually passive, innocent, and dependent on their partner's generosity for their pleasure. Women who are assertive, confident, and knowledgeable are called "sluts," and are labeled as "undesirable" or "damaged goods." What this means is, women who take pleasure into their own hands—literally or figuratively— threaten the status quo that, traditionally, insists women must be meek and dependent.

What's more, many women have been told, explicitly or implicitly, that their genitals are dirty, smelly, and ugly. So it's hardly surprising that women who have internalized this message resist touching themselves. And to make matters worse, intercourse with a partner's penis is considered the purest form of pleasure, even though it doesn't often fulfill a woman's diverse sexual needs. There's also the assumption that women who masturbate are either too unattractive to find a partner or are in unsatisfying relationships. Even though most of these beliefs usually remain unspoken, the ideas and assumptions behind them are still subtly yet pervasively present as subtexts within pop culture. They can become so ingrained in our minds that we don't even notice them until we start talking about them—*if* we talk about them—because discussing masturbation or sexuality with friends or a partner can be regarded as inappropriate or taboo. In fact, women are discouraged from touching themselves in so many ways that it's a wonder that 90 percent of women actually *have* pleasured themselves!

Think about your own experience, and reflect on what may be holding you back from touching yourself. Would you admit that you masturbate to a close friend (even if you were to leave out all the juicy details)? A lover? A therapist? If your answer is no, your reasons for holding back your admission may point to the roadblocks that are preventing you from fully embracing solo sex. The bottom line, though, is that no one should feel ashamed of touching herself: It's something to be celebrated and encouraged.

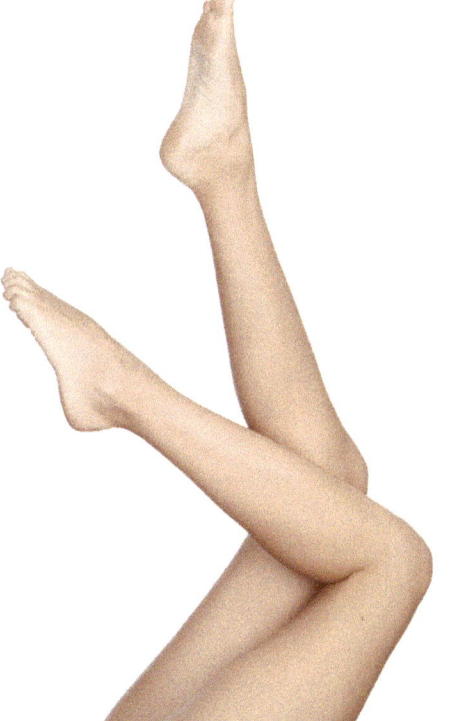

SEVEN WAYS TO FEEL GOOD ABOUT SELF-PLEASURE

1. TALK TO YOUR FRIENDS. Don't be shy—you won't offend them! Lots of your friends are self-pleasuring and can share their experiences with you.

———

2. OPEN UP TO YOUR PARTNER. He or she is probably enjoying solo sex as well, and will love that you're ready to self-explore.

———

3. LISTEN TO THE STATISTICS. Solo sex isn't an anomaly. The fact is, the overwhelming majority of women do it: 92 percent of women pleasure themselves, and two-thirds of them do it three times per week.

———

4. CONSULT YOUR DOCTOR. You may feel more relaxed and open to self-pleasure when you hear a medical professional tell you that masturbation is healthy.

———

5. REVIEW THE HEALTH BENEFITS of solo sex in chapter 1. It's great for your physical and psychological health!

———

6. FAKE IT 'TIL YOU MAKE IT. Keep doing it, even if it makes you emotionally uneasy at first. That's okay: it might take a while before your body memory recognizes it as a positive experience.

———

7. READ OTHER WOMEN'S EXPERIENCES in books or online. Hearing other women's stories of self-pleasure will normalize it for you.

———

Fortunately, sex-positive activists have spent years debunking these negative ideas about women's sexuality and self-pleasure. The feminist movement has also empowered women to take charge of their own bodies, and to transform the "shaming" narrative about sexually confident women into an inspiring, exciting one. Activists like these have shown the world that solo pleasure is natural, healthy, and beneficial to both the individual and her relationships with others. Activist Betty Dodson, for instance, wrote a book called *Liberating Masturbation* (now titled *Sex for One: The Joy of Self-Loving*), which has helped thousands of people understand, accept, and celebrate the beauty of their own bodies and their erotic responses.

USE A MANTRA

Despite the good work that's been done by the amazing women and men who are working to change the discourse surrounding self-pleasure, negative cultural messages regarding masturbation can be deep-seated and hard to budge. It's possible that, consciously and intellectually, you believe that solo sex is perfectly normal and healthy—but each time you go to touch yourself, you react with shame-filled body language and can't fully enjoy the pleasurable sensations that come with solo sex. That's because you've internalized those negative messages, and they're undermining your physiological response to pleasure. But you can counteract these negative thoughts and replace them with affirmative ones, and one way to do that is to use a mantra. When you use a mantra, you repeat the belief you want to absorb over and over again to yourself.

The classic mantra for meditation is "ohm," but in this instance, you might want to choose a mantra that speaks to pleasure—one that feels empowering (and not hokey) to you. If, when you masturbate, the negative voices in your head say, "This is dirty," counteract them with a phrase like, "Pleasure is healthy." Or if those voices are telling you you're ugly or unattractive, try a mantra like "My body is beautiful" or "My body is sacred." Tailor your mantra to your own needs and choose a phrase that feels right to you and gives you confidence. Repeat it with every outbreath, either out loud or silently. Soon those negative thoughts will fade into oblivion.

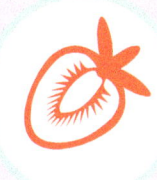

HOW CAN I RELAX?

Beat tension and get ready to enjoy your solo sexual adventures! Here's how:

———

ZONE OUT.
Get a massage, do some gardening, go for a run, stretch, play with your pet, or meditate. Do whatever puts you in tune with your body and helps you stay in the present moment—it's a great precursor to pleasure.

———

PAMPER YOURSELF.
Spend a little extra and allow yourself the fancy body lotion, the sensual bath oil, the manicure, the deluxe sex toy, or the sexy outfit. It's worth it: Treating yourself to just one special thing can help you enjoy private sexy time that much more.

———

HAVE A DRINK.
Singular, not plural. One drink can help you relax. More than two—at the very most—numbs the pleasure and becomes counterproductive.

SET ASIDE THE TIME.
If you're not convinced that this is time well spent, you'll constantly be distracted by thoughts of the "more important" things that you "should" be doing right now. Give this time to yourself, and value it: It's just as important as your other responsibilities.

———

FIND SOME PRIVACY.
Lock the door, turn off your phone, get the kids out of the house, hop into the bath—do whatever it takes to ensure that no one will disturb you.

———

DITCH THE DISTRACTIONS.
Get rid of the laundry and turn up the music so you can't hear the kids, the neighbors, or the construction that's going on outside your window—or better yet, go somewhere else. That way, you won't start planning your next renovation project or notice all the chores that need to be done. They can wait!

———

BREATHE DEEPLY.
It sounds simple, but it's true: breathing is central to relaxing and de-stressing. Remember to breathe deeply throughout the day, and especially during your solo-pleasure time. It's easy to forget, so some people even stick a Post-it note in a strategic location (like on the bathroom mirror) as a reminder!

TRY PROGRESSIVE RELAXATION.
Squeeze all of the muscles in your feet and toes for five seconds, then relax them for five seconds. Work your way up your body, repeating the process with your calves, thighs, pelvis, butt, chest, arms, and head. It only takes two minutes, and you'll feel so much more relaxed.

———

FOCUS ON THE POSITIVE.
And there are always plenty of positives. If you start to get self-critical, think about your achievements and your kindnesses toward other people and animals; think about what you love about your body; think about what you're grateful for in life. Or repeat your personal mantra to yourself. Devote a full breath to each thought, and breathe it through your entire being.

———

KEEP A NOTEBOOK ON HAND.
If brilliant ideas or things you forgot pop into your mind when it's empty, keep a notebook nearby so you can quickly jot down your thoughts and then get back to the business of pleasure.

INITIATING SELF-SEX

Planning a hot date with yourself? Start by enjoying your entire body. Indulge all of your senses: Spend half an hour in a luxurious bath, lavish yourself with your favorite scented lotion, treat yourself to a decadent snack, like a little good chocolate or some fresh fruit. Fill the space you're in with music, scents, visuals, and tastes that nourish your erotic sensibilities. Try not to rush: Take your time, because staying relaxed is the key to arousal. (If you're stressed out, chances are you'll be too worked up and distracted to feel aroused at all!)

Maybe you feel sexy or horny on a regular basis, and love touching yourself and your partner whenever you can. When you have a crush on someone or embark on a new relationship, you may feel this desire even more often. You might think about sex a lot more: remembering the last kiss, touch, or hot date; dreaming about what you'd do if you had sex right now; or plotting an X-rated surprise for next time. This

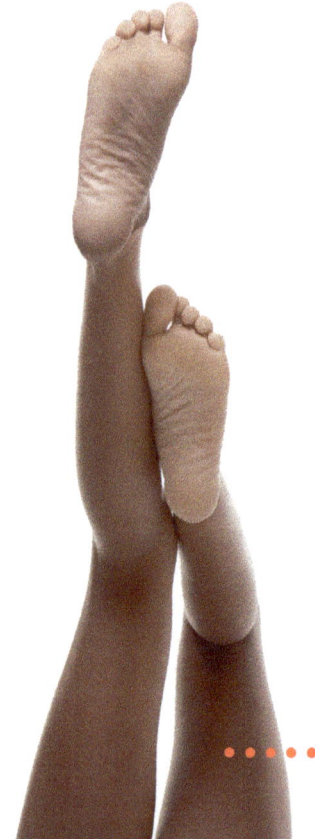

"New Relationship Energy" (NRE) is what fuels much of the high sex drive that accompanies the beginning of a new relationship. Still, you might not have experienced this intense energy—even if you have a fantastic crush on someone. Or perhaps you found yourself wanting more sex at another time in your life, but aren't up for it as regularly these days. That's fine! Everyone's sex drive is different. That said, it's easy to wonder whether your lower sex drive means there's something wrong with you—

especially when you're in a relationship with someone who craves sex regularly, or if you have friends who enjoy sex and discuss it a lot.

The truth is that there's probably nothing at all wrong with you. Hormones can have powerful effects on your libido, and people with high estrogen levels (generally women) tend to feel less desire than people with high testosterone levels (generally men). Of course, there are plenty of exceptions to this rule, and lots of other factors can also affect desire in both men and women, including medications, emotional responses to family and romantic relationships, the menstrual cycle, breast-feeding, infertility or pregnancy, career or school situations, and overall financial and physical health. Ultimately, wherever your level of desire is, it's yours, and it's perfectly normal. But if you don't feel sexual desire regularly, you might need to trigger it by getting aroused first. That's the reverse of the way in which men often experience it, so it might sound strange at first, but once you understand that arousal can spark desire, it's so much easier to kick your libido into high gear.

What this all means is, while you may not feel horny at any given moment, horniness often follows after you become aroused. For example, you might remember an occasion when you had solo or partner sex even though you weren't really in the mood for it at first. As things began to heat up and as you started to enjoy yourself, you might have been delighted that you nudged yourself to "just do it." That's because your arousal increased your level of desire, and you craved more pleasure as the encounter continued. Now, this isn't to say that you should have sex when you don't want to. But you *can* choose to have sex when you're open to it, even if you don't feel explicitly randy at the time. Once you're on board with that, you can open yourself to sex much more often—enjoying pleasure at first and continuing if the desire kicks in, or letting go if it doesn't.

So what arouses you? Maybe it's watching an erotic film, reading a sexy story, using a vibrator, or a warm, relaxing bath complete with essential oils, candles, and music, where you've got the time and space to lather yourself up with your favorite soap. Or, if words turn you on, ask your partner to write you a lusty story—then ask them to read it to you over the phone or in a private recording. Figure out what puts you in the mood, enjoy it, and know that desire won't be far behind.

WRITE IT DOWN

If it feels right to you, consider keeping a journal of your erotic progress. Think about how you feel about solo sex now: do you feel differently than you did a few days, weeks, or months ago? Which parts of your body give you the most pleasure? When you later look back on your journal after a few months of writing, you'll be surprised at the way your values, assumptions, and self-judgments have changed over time.

WOMAN-FRIENDLY PORN

If you've never found porn arousing, you're definitely not alone. Although too many erotic films privilege heterosexual male pleasure and showcase a very limited range of body types, hot, woman-friendly porn does exist! That's where the Feminist Porn Awards come in. Initiated in 2006, these awards recognize, celebrate, and endorse films that appeal to a broader audience. Specifically, award-winning feminist porn happens when:

———

All performers get their fair share of the pleasure.

———

A greater diversity of bodies, sexual expressions, activities, and/or desires appears on screen.

———

Films are made in accordance with ethical labor practices and the active consent of the performers.

———

Films are well produced—and hot!

———

Plus, you're more likely to see real orgasms and depictions of women and trans people taking control of their own fantasies in Feminist Porn Award–winning films. And that's great because, no matter who you are, you should be able to access films that reflect your body and your desires.

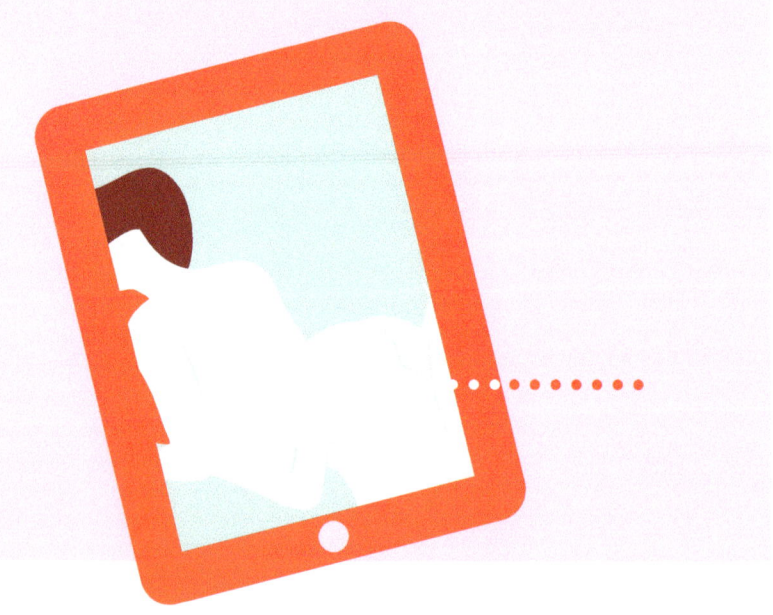

Masturbation is good for you, and now you can make it a part of your self-care routine—just like exercise or relaxation—whether you feel like having (solo) sex or not. Because you know you can get into the mood when you want to, you don't have to wait to feel sexy. Instead, you can take charge and decide that anytime is a good time to get it on—whether you're doing it with yourself or a partner.

USE IT OR LOSE IT

Just like a muscle, good habits need lots of exercise: the more you do them, the more benefits you'll reap. That's why it's important to masturbate regularly. Without frequent self-pleasure, you might find it more difficult to achieve orgasm, and sex might even become less

pleasurable in general. So make it a part of your routine: While solo sex may come easily and naturally to some people, most of us have to remember to practice it. And sometimes life gets in the way. In the same way that you avoid eating well, working out, or initiating a challenging conversation with a partner even when you know these healthy, empowering choices are good for you, it's easy to put solo sex on the back burner—only to forget about it completely. But when you *do* practice these healthy habits, you usually feel fantastic: proud, pleased, and

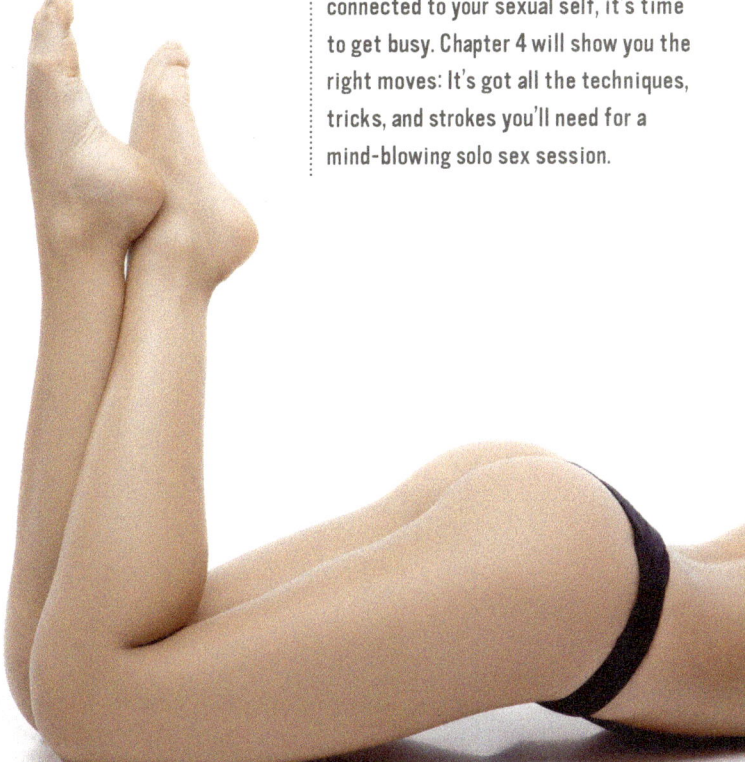

satisfied with yourself. It may have been hard to take the first step, but you're usually so glad you did.

Now that you know what arouses you (and what doesn't) and how to stay connected to your sexual self, it's time to get busy. Chapter 4 will show you the right moves: It's got all the techniques, tricks, and strokes you'll need for a mind-blowing solo sex session.

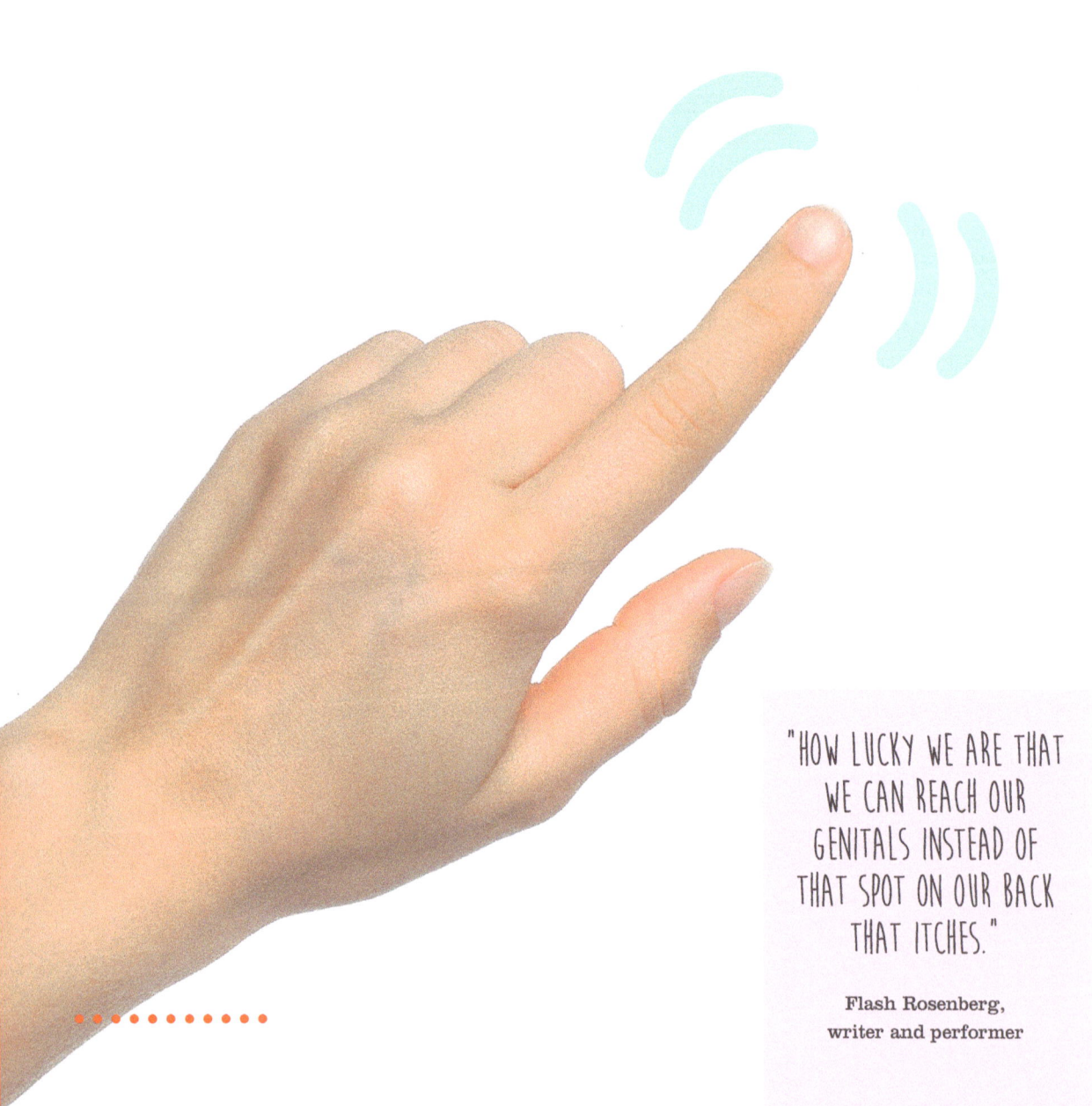

"HOW LUCKY WE ARE THAT WE CAN REACH OUR GENITALS INSTEAD OF THAT SPOT ON OUR BACK THAT ITCHES."

Flash Rosenberg,
writer and performer

HOW TO **4** SHE-BOP:
STROKES, TECHNIQUES, AND TRICKS

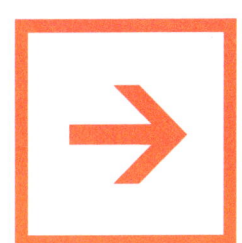

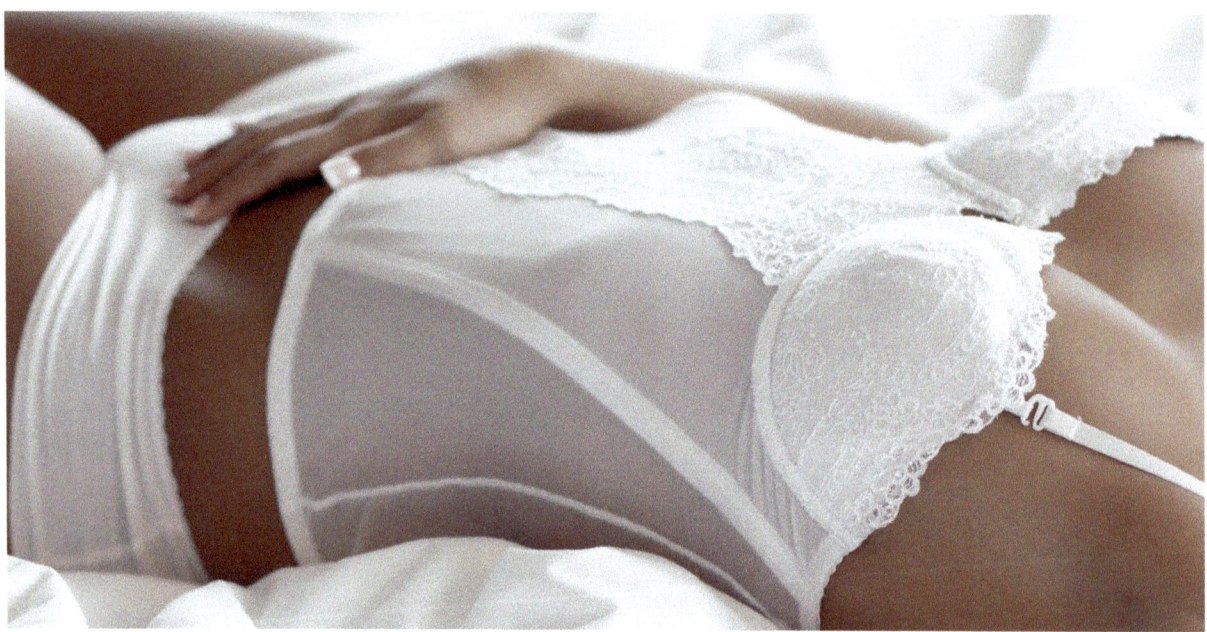

Wouldn't it be great if we were born with instruction manuals or maps that could show us everything we needed to know about our bodies? Unfortunately, evolution hasn't quite gotten there yet, so most of us begin learning about solo sex and sexual pleasure through simple trial and error. For example, maybe you started masturbating by accident, as your hand grazed your clitoris while you were washing yourself in the bath. Or perhaps you decided to embark on a voyage of self-discovery, and explore the uncharted territory between your legs simply because it was there. Or maybe you'd always found sex unsatisfying—until your partner or a friend suggested that masturbation

might help you find out what feels good to you. However it happened for you, I bet nobody ever handed you a sexual "cookbook" of recipes to try. After all, sex is a biological act, so sexual pleasure should just come naturally—right?

No way! Sexual satisfaction depends on so much more than just biological function—and a little skill and creativity is all it takes to get you there. That's where this chapter—packed with more than twenty-five positions for clitoral, labial, vaginal, and anal solo sex—comes in. Before you start, remember that there's no right or wrong when it comes to pleasure, so experimentation is king (or queen). For instance, if you enjoy penetration, you can play on your own with dildos, vibrators, and fingers. (Even if you don't like the sensation of a penis or dildo inside you during partner sex, you may like using your fingers or a toy during solo pleasure, so think about trying it before you rule it out.) Or, if penetration doesn't do anything for you, you might love stroking your labia, pleasuring your clitoris, or exploring the sensitive areas in and around your anus. Whichever way you like it, sexual pleasure is completely unique: yours won't look exactly like anyone else's. And that's the beauty of it! Let's get started.

DOS AND DON'TS OF PLEASURE

EXPERIMENT. You might be surprised as to what feels great. And sometimes what was boring five years ago ends up being amazing today!

———

TRUST YOURSELF. Don't do anything that doesn't feel good or that you don't feel comfortable doing. And just because a particular technique thrills someone else doesn't mean it will necessarily also be pleasurable for you.

———

USE LUBE. Lube is essential for most of us for great sex. Even if your vagina produces enough natural lubricant when you're aroused, it's likely that you'll still want to apply it to external areas like your clitoris, labia, anus, or perineum.

———

PAIN DOESN'T EQUAL GAIN. If it hurts, stop and try something different. Add some lube, relax, and play with a different area.

———

KEEP IT CLEAN. Don't put anything in your anus and then in your vagina (or along your vulva) without sterilizing it first. Only non-vibrating silicone toys can be sterilized in boiling water; use a condom on toys made of all other materials if you plan to use them both anally and vaginally.

———

LUBRICANTS FOR GREAT SOLO PLAY

Before you start to self-stimulate, be sure to lube up first, because lubricant makes just about any kind of sex play feel better. It's true that your vagina produces its own lubrication, which makes vaginal stimulation feel pleasurable, but you might need a little extra to provide the gliding sensation that feels so good. In general, the more aroused you are, the wetter you'll be, but a number of other factors can affect your natural lubrication levels. Many medications, such as antihistamines, can dry you out, so always research the side effects of any meds you take regularly. If oral dryness is one of them, you're likely to experience vaginal dryness as well. And hormone levels can also be a cause: If you're breast-feeding, menopausal, or at a point in your menstrual cycle other than ovulation, you're likely to be less wet. Being nervous, being dehydrated, or consuming more than a moderate amount of alcohol can also reduce your natural vaginal lubrication. And then there is just the simple fact that we are all different: Some of us can run fast and some can't. Some of us lubricate a lot, and others don't. Thankfully, lube is an easy solution!

Plus, even if you're wet inside, remember that not all sex play takes place inside the vagina. External areas like the vulva, clitoris, and anus produce no natural lubrication at all. (And natural vaginal lubricant dries out really quickly when it's exposed to air.) So you'll probably want to add some lube to your solo sex adventures, especially if you're using toys and you start playing with them before you're fully aroused.

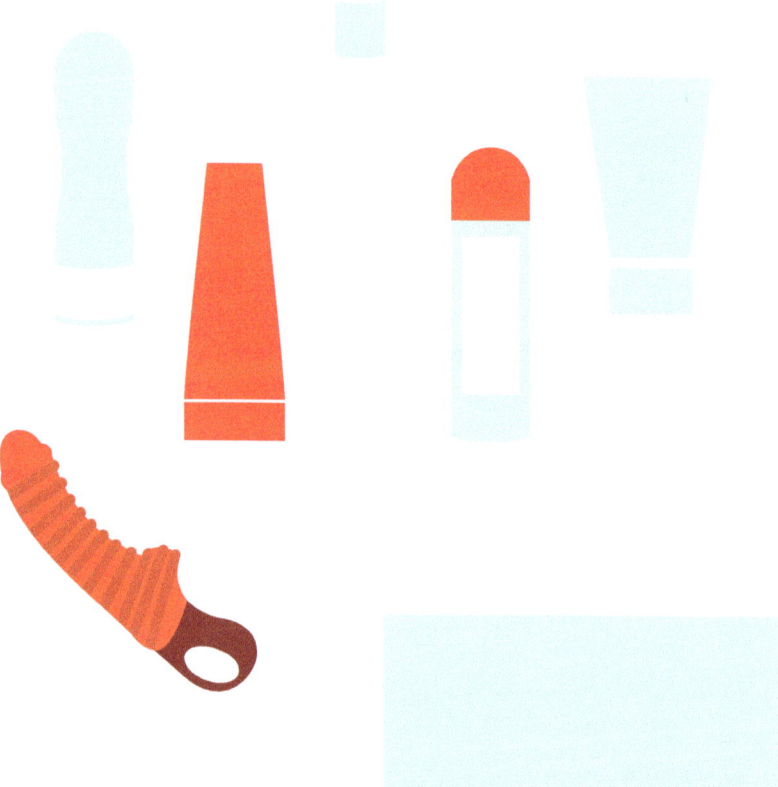

CHOOSING A LUBRICANT

Just like ice cream flavors, lube choices are really individual. Your best friend might love pistachio, but you go crazy over mint chocolate chip; in the same way, one person's favorite lube might not suit another. And you might have to try a few before you figure out which type works best for you. Some sexuality stores have tester bottles of lube, so that you can squeeze a little onto your fingers and figure out whether you like it before you buy it. Some shops even sell lubricants in single-use trial sizes: Think about buying a few and playing with them at home, because a lube might feel differently below the belt than it does on your fingers and hands. Here's a quick rundown on lubricant types.

OIL-BASED. The good news about oil-based lubricants is, they feel fabulous and last for a long time. The bad news is, you can't use them with silicone, latex, or plastic toys (or latex condoms, if you use them to cover your toy), because oil will degrade the material very quickly. You may also contract urinary tract infections (UTIs) from oil-based lubes, because the oil traps bacteria and makes it harder for your body to flush it out. If you do go for an oil-based lube, try one that's made with coconut oil, which is mildly antibacterial and might be less likely to trigger a UTI than petroleum-based oils. Use at your own risk, though!

WATER-BASED. Most of the lubes you see on store shelves are water-based, so they're safe for use with all toys. That said, not all water-based lubes are created equal and they vary in terms of how long they last, ingredients and body safety, stickiness or texture, thickness, and taste. Speaking of taste, keep in mind that flavored lubes generally dry out quickly, and it's best to apply them to a body part that can easily be licked clean. (And unless you're incredibly flexible, that's probably going to be a partner's body, not your own!)

SILICONE-BASED. These premium lubes are popular because they're so long-lasting—and that means you won't need to reapply them again and again, even if you use them externally or if your body doesn't produce much natural lubrication of its own. Silicone-based lubricants are unlikely to irritate sensitive skin, and they even stay put underwater, so they're great for use in the shower, tub, or Jacuzzi. Their only disadvantage is, silicone-based lubricants aren't compatible with many silicone toys. Test a little of the lube on an inconspicuous part of your toy. If it feels tacky or starts to discolor within one minute, it isn't compatible. Try Pjur Original, an odorless, tasteless silicone lubricant that works with many better-quality silicone toys.

WHAT'S IN MY LUBE?

Glycerin (also known as glycerol). A common lubricant ingredient, glycerin is a compound that acts like a sugar, which means two things: it gets sticky when it dries out, and it can trigger yeast infections in some women. Most flavored lubricants contain glycerin.

———

Parabens. These preservatives turn up in lots of body-care products—including lubricants— and appear under various names, such as methylparaben. Parabens have been linked to cancer in some studies, so many people prefer to avoid lubes that contain them.

———

Aloe vera. Many natural lubricants contain aloe vera, which won't cause yeast or bacterial infections and is an excellent moisturizer. Try Good Clean Love: it's a vegan, organic aloe lube that's made without glycerin or parabens.

———

Carrageenan. A seaweed extract, carrageenan has been used as a food additive for hundreds of years. These days, some studies are investigating its potential to inhibit the transmission of HPV.

———

Warming, cooling, and stimulating ingredients such as propylene glycol, alcohol, cinnamon, menthol, or peppermint oil. It might sound counterintuitive, but these ingredients actually irritate your body's sensitive tissues in order to focus your attention on that area. Some people love the sensations these additives offer, and claim that it intensifies their orgasms, while others find they yield a not-so-sexy burning sensation. If you want to try a lube with some of these ingredients, try this "progressive" approach: dab a little on your inner wrist and wait a few minutes. If that feels okay, dab a little on your thigh, then on your outer labia, and finally, on your inner labia. That way, you'll know how your body reacts to the lube before you put it on your clitoris, or inside your vagina or anus.

———

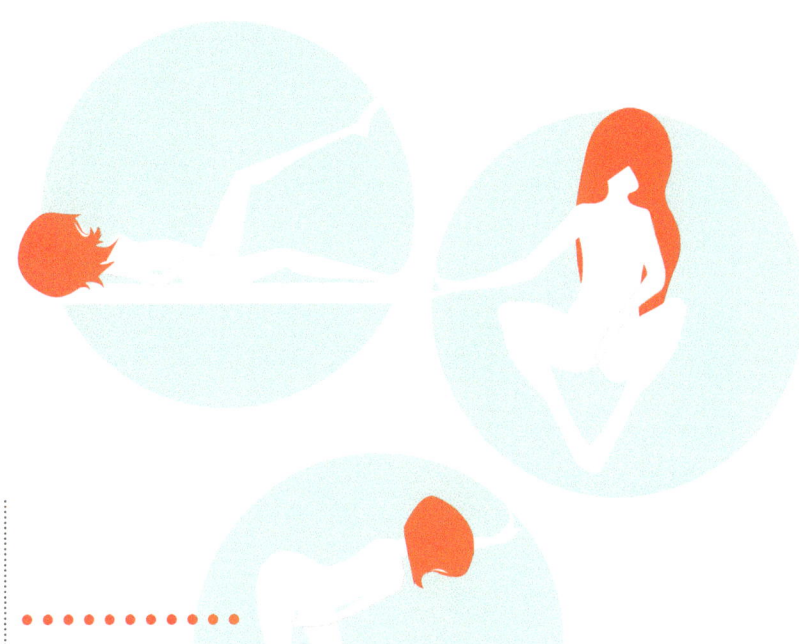

POSITIONS

You've got your favorite lube on hand and you're in the mood for a little solo sex romp, so the first thing to do is make yourself comfortable. You'll probably find that lying on your back is the easiest and most comfortable way to pleasure yourself, whether it's in your bed, on the couch, on the floor, in a field of tall grass, or in the bathtub. From that position, you can bring your knees up to your chest in a variation of the "fetal" position, if you like (anal play, for example, is easier from this angle). Or you can:

» LIE ON YOUR SIDE, either stretched out with one leg bent at a right angle, or with both legs bent in the fetal position.

» LIE ON YOUR BELLY. It can be hard to move your hands or a toy freely in this position, but it's great for moving your body up and down or grinding against a toy as if you were on top during intercourse.

» SIT in the tub or on a chair or couch, or propped against a tree, headboard, or wall.

» KNEEL. In this fun variation, you can crouch down on all fours over a toy as if you were on top during intercourse. Sit back on your heels to relax for a short time, if you want, but stop before you get pins and needles. Or sit up and brace yourself against a headboard, wall, or the back of a chair. This position is pretty challenging, though, because it takes a bit of physical effort to hold yourself up, and that can distract you from relaxing into pleasure and orgasm.

» STAND UP in the shower, in front of a mirror, in the middle of your bedroom floor—anywhere you like, really! If you need to, lean against a wall to help keep yourself from falling over when the going gets good!

How Do Women Actually Masturbate?

Sexologist Alfred Kinsey's research showed that women masturbate in lots of different ways. Here are the places that women stimulate during solo pleasure:

———

84 percent clitoris and labia

———

20 percent vaginal insertion

———

11 percent breast stimulation

———

10 percent thigh squeezing

———

5 percent muscular tension

———

2 percent fantasy alone

———

11 percent other techniques

———

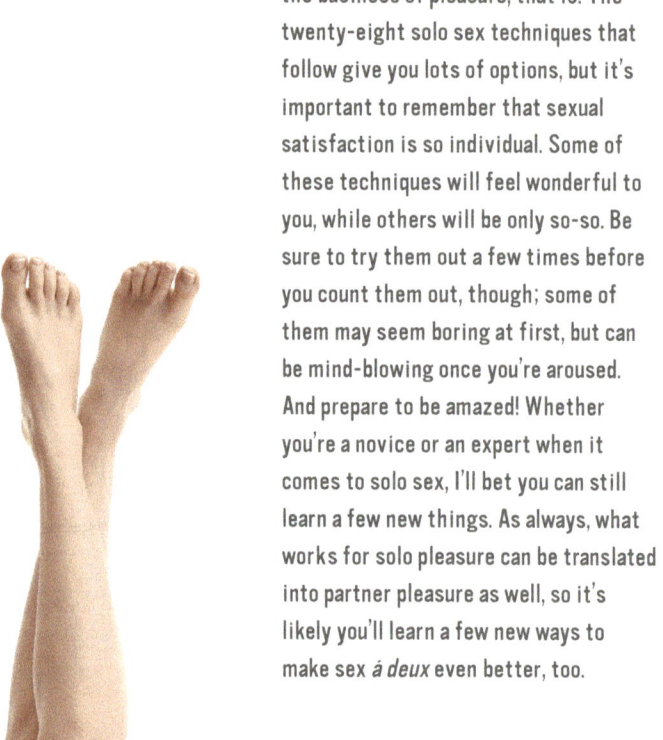

Now it's time to get down to business—the business of pleasure, that is! The twenty-eight solo sex techniques that follow give you lots of options, but it's important to remember that sexual satisfaction is so individual. Some of these techniques will feel wonderful to you, while others will be only so-so. Be sure to try them out a few times before you count them out, though; some of them may seem boring at first, but can be mind-blowing once you're aroused. And prepare to be amazed! Whether you're a novice or an expert when it comes to solo sex, I'll bet you can still learn a few new things. As always, what works for solo pleasure can be translated into partner pleasure as well, so it's likely you'll learn a few new ways to make sex *à deux* even better, too.

CLITORAL/NON-PENETRATIVE MOVES

Get ready for some serious pleasure! Here are seventeen ways to stroke, press, grind, and tease your way to great solo sex.

STROKE OF PLEASURE

POSITION: On your back or side; sitting, kneeling, or standing

TECHNIQUE: Keep your hand flat and rest it gently against your vulva. Stroke your whole hand upward, moving your hand up toward your pubic mound with fingers grazing your vulva and then over your clitoris. Lift your hand off and move it back down to the cover your whole vulva, and repeat.

VARIATIONS/ADVANCED TECHNIQUE: Use both hands, alternating them each time you stroke. Reverse the direction, moving your hand from the top of your pubic mound down (through your pubic hair, if you have any) toward your vulva.

SUGGESTIONS: Mix up the textures! Instead of your hand, use a scarf, feather, disposable latex glove, Mardi Gras beads, and any other highly textured object that you think might feel good. (See chapter 6 for options.)

WAKING UP

POSITION: On your back, side, or belly; sitting, kneeling, or standing

TECHNIQUE: It couldn't be simpler: just place your whole hand over the entire vulva, and gently shake.

VARIATIONS/ADVANCED TECHNIQUE: Apply pressure as you shake (as though you're grinding on the dance floor); undulate your hand from fingertips to heel, like a wave; use a vibrator on low power against your vulva and shake it gently.

TREAD LIGHTLY

POSITION: On your back or side; sitting, kneeling, or standing

TECHNIQUE: Graze the labia very gently with a well-lubed finger. Start at the bottom of the inner labia, and move your finger along it toward the top. Move your finger back down, and repeat.

VARIATIONS/ADVANCED TECHNIQUE: Use two fingers, one on each side of your labia, going in tandem or opposite directions. Or slow down the motion so that the stroke lasts 10 seconds. Reverse the motion, and move your finger or fingers from top to bottom, or move up and down slowly with the same hand.

BULB MASSAGE

POSITION: On your back, side, or belly; sitting, kneeling, or standing

TECHNIQUE: Use both well-lubed index fingers to massage the vestibular bulbs under the surface of the skin. (Remember that they're located just on the outside of the inner labia.)

VARIATIONS/ADVANCED TECHNIQUE: Move your fingers in alternating directions. Or spread your index and middle fingers as if you were making a peace sign, then place the "peace sign" on your vulva, with the inner labia between them. Replace one or both fingers with a vibrator (or two).

SUGGESTIONS: Try different levels of pressure; some people prefer firmer pressure, while others love a gentler touch.

LABIA ROLL

POSITION: On your back, side, or belly; sitting, kneeling, or standing

TECHNIQUE: Grab onto one of your inner labia with your thumb and index finger and roll it between your fingers, as you would roll a pen.

VARIATIONS/ADVANCED TECHNIQUE: Try grasping different parts of the labia, depending on their shape (if you have larger and longer labia, you'll be at an advantage here!). Or use both hands and massage both labia at the same time.

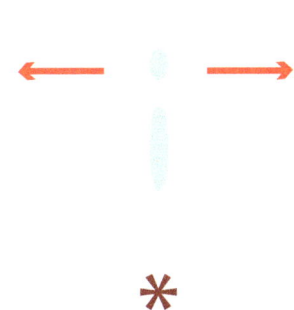

OPEN THE CUPBOARDS

POSITION: On your back or side; sitting, kneeling, or standing

TECHNIQUE: Grasp each of your inner labia with the thumb and index finger of each hand (as in the Labia Roll, above) and gently pull the labia apart.

VARIATIONS/ADVANCED TECHNIQUE: As you're grasping the labia, move them up and down or from side to side. Get creative: you can move them in different directions, if you like. Each movement yields a slightly different sensation!

SUGGESTIONS: Combine Open the Cupboards with the Labia Roll, above, for even more fun: some women find that a lot of labia movement transfers to the attached hood and thus gently stimulates the clitoris, causing plenty of good vibrations.

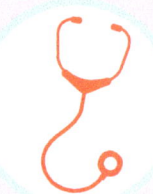

SEXSOMNIA?

It might sound strange, but it's true: some people are able to perform sexual acts while asleep, including masturbation, touching a partner, and even full-on intercourse. Sexsomnia, a recognized medical condition, is similar to sleepwalking, in which the brain is partially asleep and partially awake. Unless the sexsomniac wakes up in the process, she or he often won't remember what happened. Sexsomnia isn't necessarily a bad thing: some otherwise non-orgasmic women have reported waking up while having an orgasm in their sleep!

THREE-FINGER MASSAGE

POSITION: On your back or side; sitting, kneeling, or standing

TECHNIQUE: Start by covering your whole vulva with three well-lubed middle fingers of one hand. The tip of your middle finger will start by covering the opening to your vagina. The index and ring fingers are beside but against the vestibular bulbs, fingers spread almost as though you were indicating the number three (without worrying about moving your thumb and pinky). As you bring your hand up toward your pubic mound, your middle finger will slide right up the middle of your vulva, to your clitoris. Your index and ring fingers, trailing beside the middle finger, will massage the vestibular bulbs (as in the Bulb Massage, above) on either side of the inner labia.

VARIATIONS/ADVANCED TECHNIQUE: Gradually apply more pressure as your fingers move up toward the clitoris.

SUGGESTIONS: Some women like it when this stroke stimulates the underside of the clitoris, while others find it too intense. If you find it too full-on, just let your middle finger lift off or graze over the top of the head of the clitoris.

TAPPING

POSITION: On your back or side; sitting, kneeling, or standing

TECHNIQUE: There's just one step to this move: Gently tap your vulva with a finger, or with your whole hand.

VARIATIONS/ADVANCED TECHNIQUE: Tap just the clitoris or the shaft of the clitoris. Fold a string of plastic Mardi Gras beads against the clitoris and tap gently, and see how your body reacts to the change in texture.

SQUEEZE TEASE

POSITION: On your back or side; sitting, kneeling, or standing

TECHNIQUE: Place both hands on the outside of the vulva. Let each hand rest against a thigh, with your thumbs up above the pubic mound. Move your hands together and allow the outer and inner labia to get "squished" between the two hands, forcing the labia to pop out between your hands. Once your two hands are as close together as they can be, move them up and down slightly in alternate directions, massaging the deeper erectile tissue underneath.

VARIATIONS/ADVANCED TECHNIQUE: For more intense stimulation, replace one hand with a powerful vibrator, such as the Original Magic Wand (formerly known as the Hitachi). Be sure to place the head of the vibrator closer to the opening of the vagina than to the clitoris so as to not overwhelm you with too much intensity.

FIGURE EIGHT

POSITION: On your back or side; sitting, kneeling, or standing

TECHNIQUE: Using a well-lubed index finger, trace a figure eight. Start by drawing a little circle around the head of the clitoris, across both the inner labia and the urethra (or U-spot), and then move down and around the vaginal opening in a larger circle.

VARIATIONS/ADVANCED TECHNIQUE: Mix up the speed of the strokes: move your fingers slower or faster, or make the figure eights smaller or larger. Or try using a vibrator to trace the same pattern.

*

WINDSHIELD WIPER

POSITION: On your back, side, or belly; sitting, kneeling, or standing

TECHNIQUE: Point your well-lubed index finger downward, and run it back and forth over the hood of your clitoris like a windshield wiper, feeling the clitoral shaft underneath.

VARIATIONS/ADVANCED TECHNIQUE: Depending on your sensitivity levels, place your finger closer to or farther away from the head of your clitoris. Vary the pressure from light to heavy, and the speed from slow to fast. Change the position of your finger so that it's perpendicular to your body and the shaft of the clitoris (that is, it should be pointing sideways) and continue the same stroke, moving your finger back and forth from the side. Or replace your finger with your showerhead, and perform the same motion with water pressure. You can also use a vibrator instead of your finger.

SUGGESTIONS: Don't rush: be sure to give this technique some time. It often takes more than a minute for the pleasure to build up noticeably.

THE HER-JOB

POSITION: On your back, side, or belly; sitting, kneeling, or standing

TECHNIQUE: Using a thumb and index finger, grab onto the shaft of the clitoris over the top of the hood and massage it up and down, as though you're giving a hand job to a small penis.

VARIATIONS/ADVANCED TECHNIQUE: Try to stimulate the underside of the clitoral shaft (unless you find it too sensitive) by pinching your two fingers together from the top around to underneath the shaft. Rather than moving your fingers up and down in tandem, move your index finger up as you move your thumb down and in the reverse direction, as if you were adjusting a manual radio dial (the old-fashioned kind!). You can also use two index fingers (one finger on each side) instead. Or use a vibrator with two prongs, such as the JimmyJane Form 2, to perform the Her-Job.

SUGGESTIONS: Go gently at first, but don't be afraid to ramp up the pressure if you're not feeling much. The shaft of the clitoris can often take—and appreciate—a fair bit of pressure.

ROCK AND ROLL

POSITION: On your back, side, or belly; sitting, kneeling, or standing

TECHNIQUE: Place your index fingers on either side of the clitoris, with palms facing down. Now, the index finger of one hand *rocks up and down* against the side of the shaft of the clitoris, while the index finger of the other hand *rolls around* in a circle against the shaft.

VARIATIONS/ADVANCED TECHNIQUE: Switch hands, so that the rocking side now rolls, and the rolling side now rocks. Or try this technique with different fingers from both hands, such as your middle finger or your ring finger. For a little extra excitement, use a vibrator instead of a hand on one side of the clitoris.

SUGGESTIONS: It's easiest to Rock and Roll if you move both of your hands in the same rhythm, so that one up-and-down "Rock" stroke has the same pace and timing as one "Roll" stroke on the other side.

AROUND THE CLOCK PLEASURE

POSITION: On your back, side, or belly; sitting, kneeling, or standing

TECHNIQUE: Using a well-lubed finger, push your clitoris in different directions, as though it were the hour hand on a clock. Try two o'clock, five o'clock, six o'clock (which involves pulling up the underside of the clitoris), nine o'clock, or twelve o'clock (pushing your clitoris straight down toward your feet).

VARIATIONS/ADVANCED TECHNIQUE: Try Around the Clock Pleasure with a vibrator on low speed instead of your finger. Or move your finger or the vibrator in small circles at each hour.

*

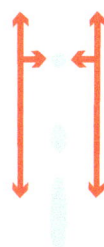

*

GOT YOUR CLIT

POSITION: On your back or side; sitting, kneeling, or standing

TECHNIQUE: This technique is a little like the game kids love to play, where you grab your thumb between your index and middle finger as you tell them, "Got your nose!" Of course, this version is all grown-up: you use the well-lubed middle and index fingers of one hand to grab your clitoris instead of your thumb. Here's how: place the back of your hand against your body, palm facing out. Run your two fingers down the sides of the shaft of the clitoris, squeezing the shaft between your fingers. As you move further down the vulva past the clitoris, focus the pressure inward against the vestibular bulbs. When you reach the lower end of your vulva, move your fingers back up again in the same way. Try to keep your arm in one place while your hand moves up and down, bending at the wrist.

VARIATIONS/ADVANCED TECHNIQUE: Apply a little more pressure as you squeeze your fingers together. Or focus the pressure on your vestibular bulbs as you move your fingers up and down. You can also shorten the stroke so that just the shaft of the clitoris gets all the stimulation.

SUGGESTIONS: If your flexibility is limited, you might find this technique difficult to do yourself. So if you've got a partner, why not bring her or him into the action?

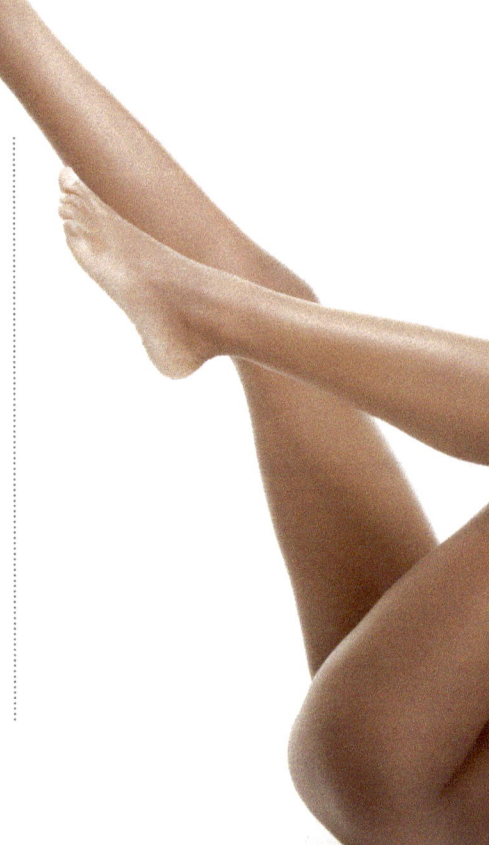

VARIATIONS/ADVANCED TECHNIQUE:

On the way back up, spread your index and middle fingers so that they run outside the inner labia and graze the vestibular bulbs.

SUGGESTIONS:
There's a lot of movement going on here, so make sure you're very well lubed!

PAINFUL SEX

If some types of stimulation on the outside or putting a finger, toy, or tampon inside your vagina feels painful, stop immediately. Forcing yourself to endure the pain will only convince your body that sex hurts, and your vagina will respond by tightening up even more every time you attempt it. Only do what feels pleasurable.

There are plenty of pleasure options, many of which don't involve penetration. Check out the book *When Sex Hurts* by Andrew Goldstein; it might help you isolate the cause of the pain. Also, consider talking to your health care provider and/or a physiotherapist about what might help you enjoy external and/or internal stimulation.

GLIDE AND TWIST

POSITION: On your back or side; sitting, kneeling, or standing

TECHNIQUE: Start with the "Got Your Clit" technique. After the downstroke, instead of moving your hand back up the same way, rotate your wrist instead so that your palm is now facing inward. Dip your index and middle fingers into the opening of the vagina, then move them back up the middle of your vulva all the way up to the shaft of the clitoris. Then, turn your hand back out so that the palm is facing out (like at the beginning of the stroke) and repeat, grabbing onto your clitoris again as you move your hand back down.

GOING IN CIRCLES

POSITION: On your back, side, or belly; sitting, kneeling, or standing

TECHNIQUE: Pull back on the hood of the clitoris (you can do this by pulling up with one hand from the pubic mound). With a well-lubed finger from your other hand, make slow, gentle circles around the head of the clitoris, or use the pressure from the showerhead instead of your finger.

VARIATIONS/ADVANCED TECHNIQUE: If you crave a more intense sensation, replace your finger with a vibrator on low speed.

SUGGESTIONS: Take your time with this one! Pleasure builds when you go extra slowly and gently here, reducing the intensity and making you much more likely to enjoy this stroke.

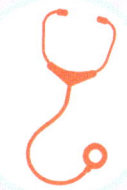

CONQUERING VAGINISMUS: BREATHE, SQUEEZE, AND RELEASE

Vaginismus—tightening of the vagina during penetration—can make penetrative sex (solo or partnered) difficult, or even impossible. But this technique can help. When you're well aroused, insert a well-lubed finger or toy (preferably thin, like a finger) into your vagina. When you feel pain, don't pull it out. Instead, keep the finger or toy still, take a deep breath, squeeze your vaginal muscles against the finger or toy for a few seconds, and then relax as you release your breath. The pain will often subside. If it does, move the finger or toy slowly again. If the pain resumes, repeat the process: breathe, squeeze, and relax. If you have been feeling pain for a while, it may take several sessions in which you use the "breathe, squeeze, and release" technique before you're able to move a finger or toy in and out without stopping. It may take as long as ten minutes for you to be able to move a finger or toy in and out just a few times. But as long as you don't force yourself to endure pain, you might find that it gets easier after a few sessions, and you may be able to move the finger or toy in and out faster, without feeling pain or stopping. Then you can graduate to moving faster or inserting two fingers or a larger toy, starting slowly and building up as you did with the single finger. This technique does require much patience—but it just might help.

VAGINAL TECHNIQUES

Lots of women find penetrative solo play really pleasurable. Here's how to start.

CIRCLES AT THE DOORSTEP

POSITION: On your back, side, or belly; sitting, kneeling, or standing

TECHNIQUE: Use one, two, or more well-lubed fingers to trace shallow circles at the opening of the vagina.

VARIATIONS/ADVANCED TECHNIQUE: Use an insertable toy instead of your fingers. Vary the speed from very slow (10 seconds per circle) to very fast. Experiment with different amounts of pressure; some women prefer a feather-light touch, while others like firm pressure. Instead of moving your fingers only, rotate your wrist as well for even more stimulation.

PERINEAL SPONGE

POSITION: On your back, side, or belly; sitting, kneeling, or standing

TECHNIQUE: Insert one thumb and push your fingers toward the back wall of the vagina (opposite the G-spot, toward your tailbone). Massage the area up and down with the pads of your thumb.

VARIATIONS/ADVANCED TECHNIQUE: Try using two fingers instead. Move your fingers or thumb back and forth, like a windshield wiper, or tap or press, as if you were ringing a doorbell. Move in circles instead of pushing, or experiment with an insertable toy.

SUGGESTIONS: First-timers, take note: it's much easier to insert a thumb than it is to insert two fingers. Plus, using your thumb makes it easier to stimulate the perineum using the index and middle fingers of the same hand on the outside at the same time.

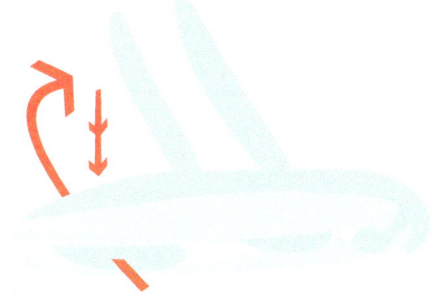

G-SPOT

POSITION: On your back, side, or belly; sitting, kneeling, or standing

TECHNIQUE: Insert two fingers, and then curl them so they're pressed up and against the front wall of the vagina. You'll probably be able to feel your pubic bone through the layers of tissue. Make a "come hither" or beckoning motion with your fingers to stimulate the G-spot.

VARIATIONS/ADVANCED TECHNIQUE: Once your fingers are inside, spread them into a peace sign and then make the "come here" motion, or try the Windshield Wiper technique, above. Try this technique with shallow penetration (just one knuckle's-depth inside) or with deep penetration (with your fingers inside as far as they'll go). Experiment with different levels of pressure. Instead of your fingers, try either a soft or firm curved toy.

SUGGESTIONS:

» **USE THE BATHROOM** before you start. If you feel like you have to pee during stimulation, breathe through it: the full-bladder sensation will usually dissipate after a few sessions as your brain begins to reinterpret the feeling as pleasurable. If you still can't relax, try playing with your G-spot in the shower—where you might be more comfortable urinating, in case an accident happens—or even while sitting on the toilet. (Many a G-spot has been found while on the toilet, because lots of people don't feel comfortable with the possibility of peeing anywhere else.)

» **WHEN YOU'RE USING A TOY** against your G-spot, pull it out instead of pushing it in. A toy with a prominent head on it—one that's a little wider than the shaft—makes this technique even more pleasurable.

» **STAY AROUSED.** Keep stimulating your clitoris (or wherever else feels good) while you look for the G-spot. If your arousal diminishes, blood will flow out of the erectile tissue and play will no longer feel pleasurable.

HOW CAN I LEARN TO SQUIRT?

LIST COURTESY OF SEX EDUCATOR TARA MCKEE. WWW.TARAMCKEE.COM

To help with that "I need to pee" sensation, go to the bathroom first.

———

Afraid of making a mess? Put down a few layers of towels (just in case).

———

Get aroused first, whichever way you like it! This makes the spot easier to find.

———

Stimulate the G-spot directly (it's on the upper vaginal wall).

———

Curled fingers or a curved toy are best. Rub them around and explore.

———

Hint: If you feel the need to pee, you've probably found it!

———

Keep going. Mix up G-spot pressure with clitoral stimulation, if you like.

———

If you feel the urge to push, go for it. This part can be tricky to figure out, so remember to relax and enjoy the stimulation.

———

You may feel pressure and pleasure building; it'll probably feel different from clitoral stimulation.

———

Some women like to take the toy or fingers out and rub them on the (external) U-spot to help them let go and squirt.

———

Fluid levels vary. Sometimes there's a little; sometimes there's a lot; and sometimes you'll just pee out the fluid later (which means it was redirected into your bladder).

———

Ejaculation can occur with or without an orgasm, or before, during, or after. Ejaculate or no ejaculate: how do you feel? Anything new and interesting?

———

A-SPOT

POSITION: On your back or side; sitting, kneeling, or standing

TECHNIQUE: The A-spot is located deeper inside than the G-spot, on the upper wall of the vagina, so you might need to use a toy in order to reach it. Soft toys made from silicone or elastomer work for some women, while others enjoy the firmer pressure delivered by harder toys made from silicone over plastic; stainless steel; wood; or glass.

VARIATIONS/ADVANCED TECHNIQUE: Try making the come-hither motion with your fingers or toy. If you're using your fingers, spread them into the peace sign, then press on the upper wall of the vagina. Play around with different pressure levels and with the depth and length of each stroke.

WHAT IS FEMALE EJACULATE?

According to Deborah Sundahl in *Female Ejaculation and the G-Spot*, the G-spot, or urethral sponge, is homologous to the male prostate. With arousal and/or orgasm, it produces a clear fluid in approximately thirty glands and emits the fluid through ducts that lead into the urethra. It is not urine. The fluid contains prostate-specific antigen (PSA), which is also produced in the male prostate. Only 15 to 20 percent of women ejaculate. Women who don't ejaculate likely have a "retrograde" ejaculation that goes into the bladder rather than exiting the body. One study found the presence of PSA in 75 percent of women's post-sex urine and no PSA in pre-sex urine. If you don't ejaculate, you may notice that your bladder is full after sex; this is the ejaculate that has gone inward and filled the bladder.

DOUBLE THE PLEASURE: G-SPOT AND CLITORIS

POSITION: On your back, side, or belly; sitting, kneeling, or standing

TECHNIQUE: Simultaneous internal and external stimulation makes for serious pleasure. Use one hand (whichever hand you feel comfortable with) to stimulate the G-spot using any of the techniques above, such as the "come hither" motion. At the same time, use your other hand to pleasure your clitoris however you like it: try Around the Clock Pleasure (page 77), for example.

VARIATIONS/ADVANCED TECHNIQUE: Finding the right combination of movements will really nudge you over the edge. So experiment: Mix your favorite style of G-spot stimulation (deeper or shallower, harder or softer, fingers together or apart) with whatever kind of clitoral stimulation gets you going (such as the Figure Eight, Her-Job, or Windshield Wiper). You can also use a vibrator in either spot—or on both at the same time!

SUGGESTIONS: If the sensation feels too intense and overwhelming, alternate: Stimulate your G-spot, then your clitoris, and then back to the G-spot, alternating every five to ten seconds.

DOUBLE UP: G-SPOT AND THE BACK-DOOR G

POSITION: On your back, side, or belly; sitting, kneeling, or standing

TECHNIQUE: Stimulate the G-spot with the fingers of one hand or a toy, and place your other hand on your lower abdomen, just above the pubic bone; press gently. This technique stimulates the G-spot from both the inside and the outside.

VARIATIONS/ADVANCED TECHNIQUE: If you don't have a sensitive bladder, go ahead and put a lot of pressure on your lower abdomen. With the fingertips of one hand on the inside and your other hand on the outside, your hands might be able to feel one another through the tissue of the vaginal wall.

SUGGESTIONS: Don't force it (and that goes for all of the techniques in this chapter!). The Double Up usually inspires a love-or-hate reaction, so if you fall into the latter category, stop and try something else. If you enjoy intercourse on a full bladder, you're more likely to appreciate this technique.

DOUBLE-DIPPING: G-SPOT AND PERINEAL SPONGE

POSITION: On your back, side, or belly; sitting, kneeling, or standing

TECHNIQUE: Use the fingers of one hand to pleasure your G-spot, located on the front wall of the vagina, while using the thumb of your other hand to stimulate the perineal sponge described on page 80.

VARIATIONS/ADVANCED TECHNIQUE: Try different depths of both hands. Alternate the movements of both hands; switch every five seconds. Replace one hand with a toy. Place the index finger of your second hand into your anus so that you can massage the perineal sponge from both the vaginal and anal sides. Or use a vibrator like the Vitality to pleasure the front and back walls of your vagina simultaneously.

DIGGING FOR PLEASURE

POSITION: On your back, side, or belly; sitting, kneeling, or standing

TECHNIQUE: Thrust inside with one or more fingers, while your thumb remains outside, bumping against your labia and clitoris.

VARIATIONS/ADVANCED TECHNIQUE: Keep your fingers together on the way in, spread them on the way out. Twist your fingers rather than pushing and pulling them straight in and out, or use a glass dildo that has a diagonal twist for the same effect. Use a soft toy for deeper cervical stimulation; angle the toy deeply toward the back for cul-de-sac pleasure.

SUGGESTIONS: Some love thrusting sensations during solo sex, but others don't enjoy doing it, even if they enjoy having intercourse with a partner. That's okay: as the saying goes, different strokes for different folks!

ANAL TECHNIQUES

If you've ever thought of exploring your back door, you're not alone. Despite being a little taboo, anal stimulation can be incredibly pleasurable! Here are a few ways to help you experiment.

TEASE THE ROSEBUD

POSITION: On your back in fetal position or on your side or belly; sitting, kneeling, or standing

TECHNIQUE: Simply use a well-lubed finger to explore the outside of the anus.

VARIATIONS/ADVANCED TECHNIQUE: Mix up the motion! Move your finger in circles; try the "doorbell" (see Perineal Sponge) or Windshield Wiper techniques mentioned above; let the tips of your fingers wiggle along the crack of your butt; or simply pull your butt cheeks apart! Put a condom on your vibrator (if you're going to use it for vaginal stimulation at another time) and run it along the outside of your anus.

GETTING THE MOST FROM ANAL PLAY

No pressure. Don't worry, penetration isn't the only thing that feels good: External anal pleasure feels great, too.

———

Stay wet. Be sure to use lubricant for any anal play.

———

Use a glove. If you're going to move your hand back to your vulva or vagina, a disposable glove makes for an easy transition (just take off the glove; no need to wash your hands in between).

———

Pain-free. Inserting a toy or fingers anally shouldn't hurt. If it does, add lube; slow down; spend more time stimulating the outside of your anus first, to warm it up; or just leave it for another time.

———

Take your time. In general, the slower you go, the more pleasure you feel.

———

Use a toy with a flared base. In fact, don't insert anything into your butt that doesn't have a flared base. The anus has a tendency to swallow toys, and you don't want your solo sex session to end with a trip to the emergency room!

———

FINGER PLAY

POSITION: On your back in fetal position or on your side or belly; sitting, kneeling, or standing

TECHNIQUE: After lots of external anal play, insert a well-lubed finger and just hold it in place without moving it.

VARIATIONS/ADVANCED TECHNIQUE: Move your finger a little, but rather than simply thrusting it in and out, try shaking your hand. That'll transform your finger into a vibrator while it's inside you. Or hold a vibrator in your palm to conduct the vibrations to your finger, then make little circles with your finger, keeping your wrist in one place. You can also twist your wrist, keeping your finger still so that the pad of your finger moves around, stimulating the sensitive tissue.

SUGGESTIONS: Stimulate your vagina and/or your clitoris at the same time for a triple-whammy of pleasure.

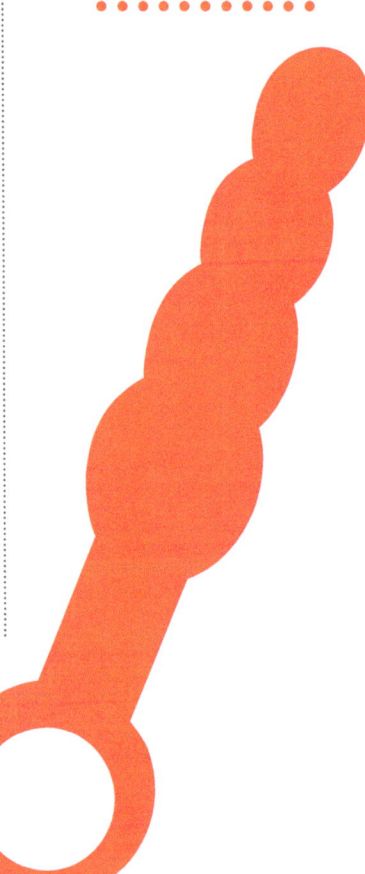

BUTT PLUG

POSITION: On your back, side, or belly; on your back in fetal position; sitting or kneeling; standing in the shower or lying in the bath

TECHNIQUE: Insert a small, well-lubed butt plug, such as the Quattro, and leave it in place.

VARIATIONS/ADVANCED TECHNIQUE: Move the outer part of the butt plug in a circle, or up and down, instead of in and out. Slowly withdraw the butt plug, then reinsert it. Play with other erogenous zones while leaving the plug in place. Or leave the plug in place while stimulating your vagina, and notice how the plug next door affects the vaginal sensations.

SUGGESTIONS: The anus has so many nerve endings that simply moving your body without touching the butt plug at all will create pleasurable sensations.

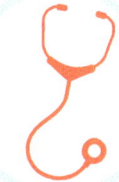

WHY CAN'T I MOVE MY FINGERS OR TOY FROM ANUS TO VAGINA?

E. coli and other bacteria live inside your butt, and these bacteria can cause vaginal or urinary tract infections. For the same reason that you're supposed to wipe from front to back, not back to front, after using the toilet, you should never move your finger or toy from your anus to your vulva or vagina without washing it thoroughly first.

Congratulations: you've done a little self-exploration, and you've learned all sorts of techniques that make for smashing solo sex! But having the right tools is as important as knowing what to do with them. Chapter 5 will show you how to choose the sex toys that can make solo pleasure even better.

BEST WORKOUT EVER

Incredibly, some women do have orgasms while they're working out! Forty-five percent of women who have experienced exercise-induced orgasms (EIOs) report that they occur during abdominal exercises, while 19 percent say that biking or spinning brings them on. Another 7 percent report that they happen during weight lifting—not to mention running, yoga, swimming, working out on elliptical machines, and other activities. Interestingly, most women said they were not fantasizing or thinking about anyone to whom they were attracted during those experiences. So what's the most popular orgasm-inducing exercise? It's the "Captain's Chair," in which you rest your weight on padded armrests while your legs hang free, then you lift your knees up toward your chest. Need any more incentive to hit the gym?

"EVEN IF TIMES ARE TOUGH
AND YOU'RE ENDURING A
TERRIBLE HEARTACHE, IT'S
IMPORTANT TO FOCUS YOUR
ANGER ON A VIBRATOR,
NOT ANOTHER PERSON."

Chelsea Handler,
*My Horizontal Life: A
Collection of One-Night Stands*

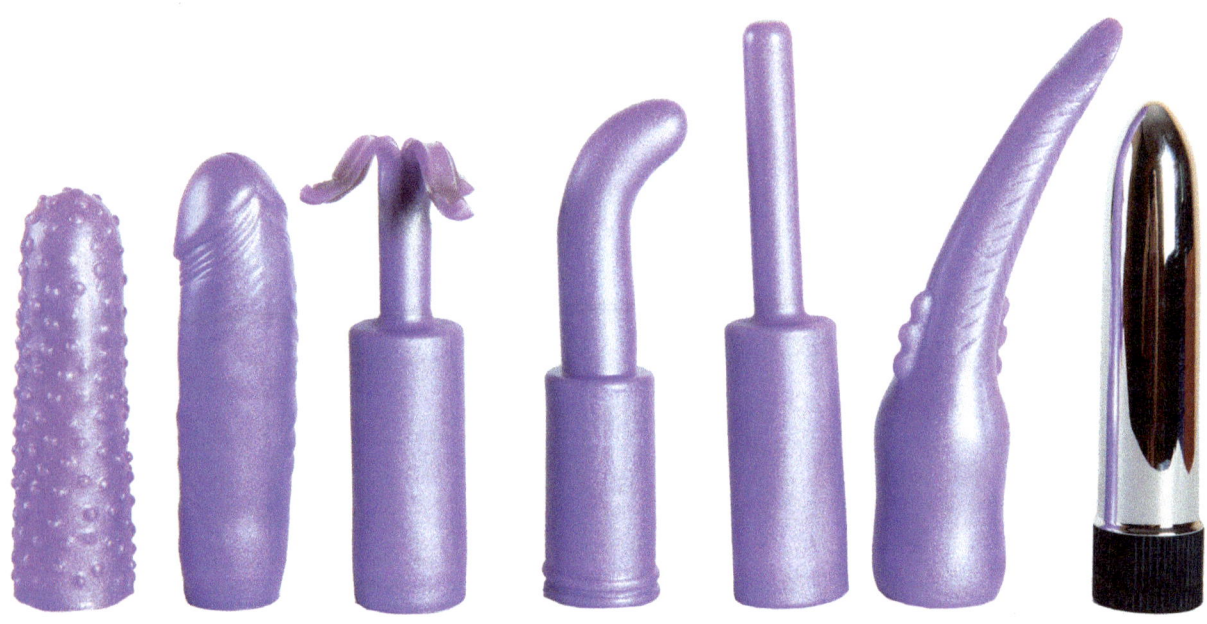

5

CHOOSING AND USING
SEX TOYS

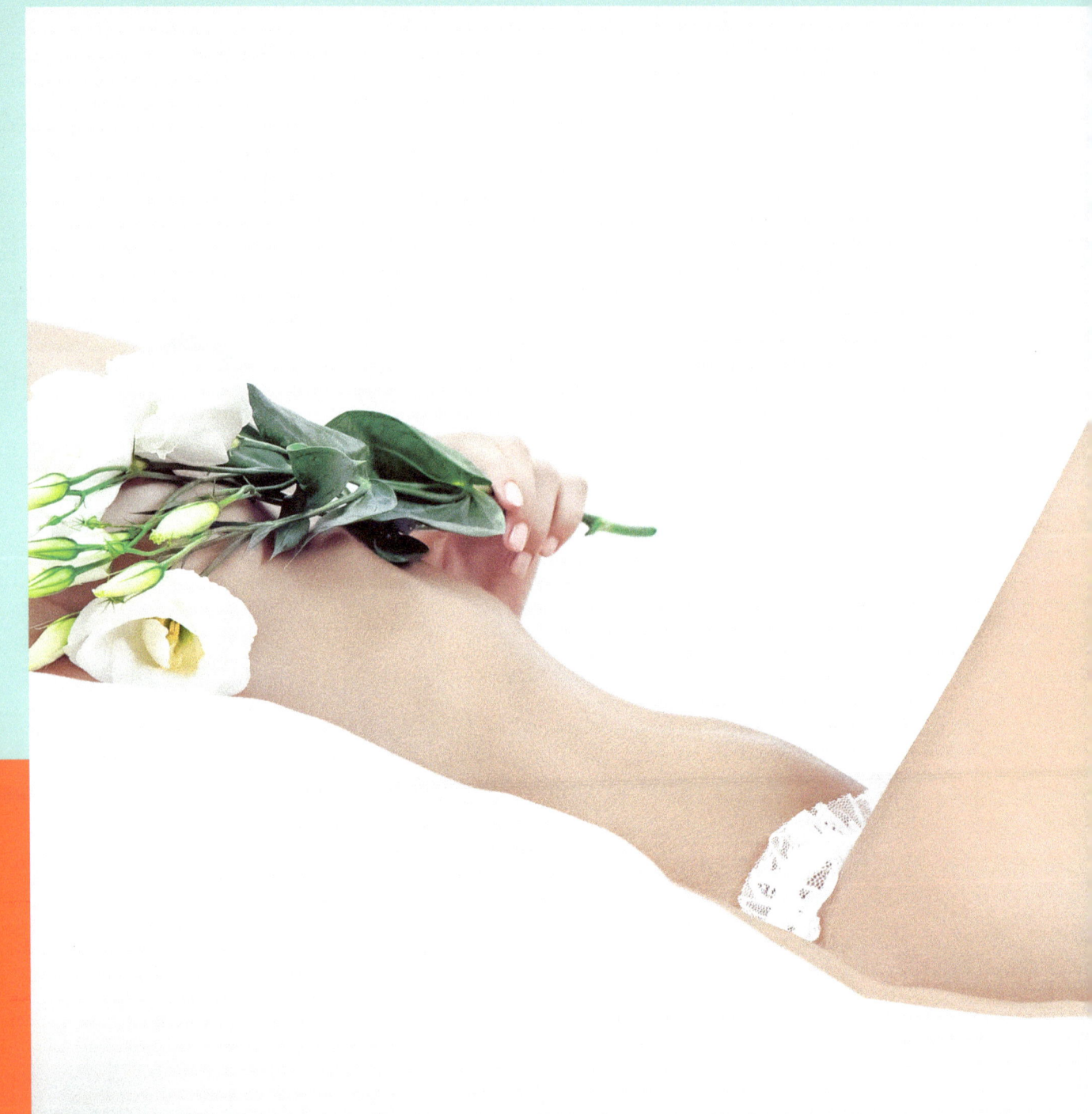

One of the best things about solo sex is that you're completely in charge of each encounter and you can do pretty much anything that feels good. Time, place, technique, fantasies, and different parts of the body, it's all up to you. Although it's possible that all you need is your own hand to rocket you into new realms of pleasure, lots of people enjoy getting a little help from wisely chosen sex toys. Why? There are lots of reasons: you may need a little extra "oomph" in order to orgasm; you might want to stimulate more hot spots than two hands can reach at a time; or perhaps it's just time for a little variety. Whatever your reasons are, you've got more options these days when it comes to sex toys than ever

before. So, even if you already have experience with toys, read on: you can't possibly have done it all, and that means that plenty of new sensations await! This chapter will help you choose the vibrators, dildos, and other sex toys that are great accessories for your solo sex adventures. (Even everyday household objects can safely double as sex toys—once you know what to do with them, that is!)

AROUND THE HOUSE

Guess what? You don't have to spend any extra cash to enjoy sex toys. Chances are, you already own a few things that can deliver a hefty dose of pleasure. Here are just a few.

WATER POWER

This one is the easiest, and it lives in your bathroom. If you have a detachable showerhead, for goodness sake, use it! Its water pressure offers unparalleled pleasure (and hey, it counts as multitasking, because you're getting clean at the same time). Aim the stream at your clitoris or anus—but don't force the flow inside. It feels amazing, and it's unlike any sensation a vibrator, finger, or tongue can ever offer. If you haven't got a detachable showerhead, try attaching a hose to the bathtub faucet: it'll produce a steady stream of water, not a spray, but it works almost as well. A Jacuzzi jet also has a powerful stream—you'll just have to execute some fancy yoga moves in order to sidle up close to the jets. It's equally as challenging to position yourself under the bathtub faucet—but if you can manage it, you'll find that a dripping tap provides a deliciously exciting rhythmic sensation. Figure out whether you prefer a slow dribble or a steadier stream, then simply lie back and enjoy.

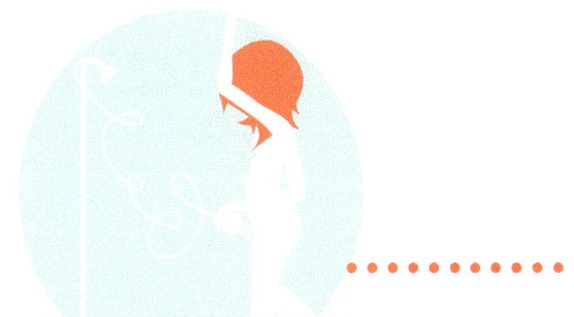

BACK AND BODY MASSAGER

You may already own a massager to help banish muscular aches and pains. While the "Original Magic Wand" is the most popular model (and for very good reasons), playing with any back or body massager is an inexpensive way to start exploring the world of sex toys. If your massager has multiple attachments, experiment to see which one feels best for you, but here's a hint: The broadest side usually yields the most pleasurable sensations. If the power is too intense for you even when your massager is set to the lowest speed, place a washcloth over your vulva to subdue the vibrations and, as in partner sex, don't go straight for the clit!

WASHING MACHINE

I know, I know, it's been done to death on TV and in the movies—but it does the trick for some people! Washing machines don't provide very intense vibration, but that suits some women. So if you can find a private moment to sit on or straddle the corner of a washing machine, give it a shot. (Suddenly, doing the laundry sounds like a lot more fun....)

ELECTRIC TOOTHBRUSH

Lots of people experiment with electric toothbrushes in their teens, when they're not legally permitted to visit sex stores—and they're a great way to start exploring! Remove the toothbrush attachment and place a condom over the shaft. Try different power settings, and enjoy a little external play (but don't put it inside you; most toothbrush shafts aren't smooth enough for internal stimulation). If you share the bathroom, be sure to remove the condom before replacing the toothbrush in its dock to avoid answering any challenging questions from housemates or family members!

GOOD VIBRATIONS

Seamstresses in the early 1900s were reported to use sewing machines to achieve orgasm by sitting near the edge of their chairs.

CELL PHONES

Giving new meaning to the phrase "ring my bell," your cell phone has a built-in vibrator. And just because it wasn't put there to get you off doesn't mean it can't be used for just that! Depending on your phone's model, you may be able to set it to vibrate constantly—very handy when it comes to solo pleasure. Use it over your underwear or put a condom over it, because you don't want your natural juices to soak into the electronic inputs or keys. (Replacing a cell phone is a lot more expensive than buying a vibrator!)

FULL-BODY TOYS

Pleasure is a full-body pursuit, and stimulating or teasing your entire body is a great way to get in the mood. If you don't already have these at home, think about investing in a couple: they probably won't cost you more than a few dollars.

» **MARDI GRAS BEADS.** These feel awesome. Dig them out of your cupboard or find them at the dollar store, because they're worth it. Drag them along the length of your body, or for an incredible tingling sensation, against your vulva. Or grasp the folded string of beads in your hand and use it to tap your vulva gently. The possibilities are endless: These things are truly worth their weight in gold.

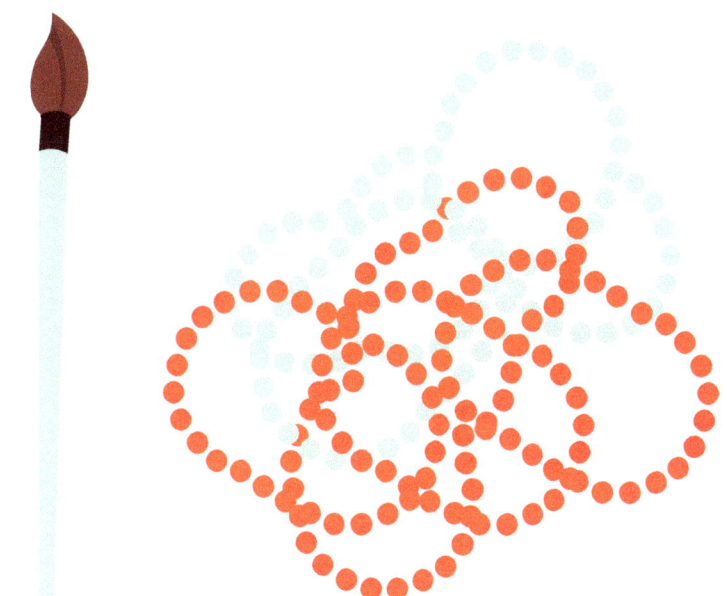

» **MASSAGE TOOLS.** Here's a good rule of thumb: If you can use it to massage somebody else, you can use it to pleasure yourself! Grab any rolling massage toy, and run it up and down your arms and legs, or roll it gently over your tummy and chest, and enjoy the soothing sensations.

» **MAKEUP BRUSHES OR PAINTBRUSHES.** Small or large, brushes can offer you a whole world of pleasure. Use brushes of different textures to stroke erogenous zones like your inner arms, tummy, nipples, inner thighs, vulva, or outer anus. (You may want to keep them separate from the paintbrushes you use for your art projects or makeup.)

» **FEATHERS.** Like brushes, feathers can be fabulously tickly. Run them over your whole body or pay special attention to your vulva or clitoris.

» **TEXTURES AND TEXTILES.** "Sensuous" starts here. Silk, leather, velvet, suede, fur (real or faux), rubber, and cotton all feel different on the skin, and you can find them in scarves, gloves, wraps, and dresses (to name a few). Don't stop there, though! If you like intense sensations, try a pick, comb, Wartenberg wheel, or anything that has a (not-too-sharp) point. Play with contrasting textures: mix and match to find out which combinations you like best.

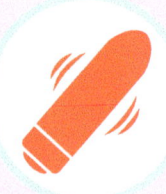

CONTRAST KEEPS IT HOT

When you're experimenting with different sensations, play with contrasting textures, pressures, and speeds: Mix fast movements with slower ones, and intense pressure with a soft, gentle touch; use a soft toy after a scratchy texture; or try following a heavy toy with a lighter object, like a feather. It's a great way to keep solo sex interesting and playful.

TREASURES FROM THE SEX TOY STORE

You've decided you want to invest in a sex toy, but what do you do when there are just so many to choose from? First things first: Get off the Internet. If there's a good sex shop in your area, visit it. It's a great way to see the products in the flesh, so to speak, and you'll get to talk to a knowledgeable staff member about which toys are right for you. Many high-quality shops also have demonstration products on display, so you can actually touch and hold each toy and get a feel for its power, quality, and ease of operation (some have finicky buttons). Check out independent stores (see Resources for a list) that value education and safely made toys, such as the Progressive Pleasure Club, a network of both brick-and-mortar and online stores in the US and Canada that are "dedicated to helping people make informed decisions about sexuality products . . . that meet the highest standards of safety." Plus, lots of independent stores like these offer fabulous workshops that can help you develop your sexual knowledge and skills. Even if you can't physically visit a sex shop, you should still call the shop and ask a staff member questions over the phone (preferably after you've done your Internet research, or even while you're doing it). That way, you'll be more likely to choose wisely. And beware of purchasing online from discount sites such as Amazon: They're full of poor-quality knock-offs, and even educated consumers have been known to make choices they've regretted. Shop small and local instead: It's good for your community, your body, and your conscience.

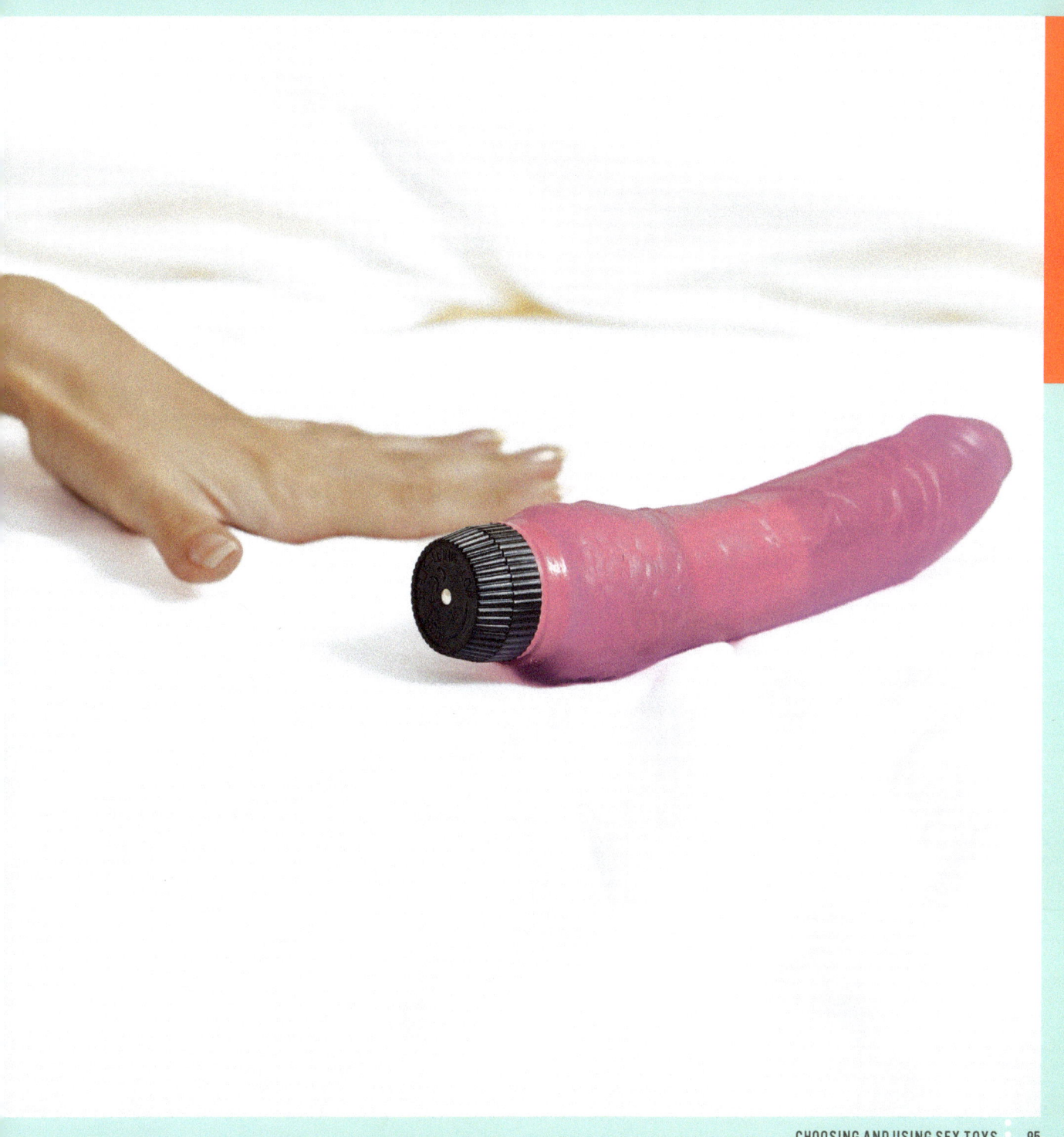

Before you invest in the sex toy of your dreams, think about these factors:

POWER. If you have a hard time orgasming, you'll probably prefer a toy with a lot of power, because the extra vibrations can help nudge you over the edge. If you're easily orgasmic, though—that is, if you can bring yourself to orgasm with your fingers within 10 minutes—you may prefer less power. In that case, also make sure that a toy's low speed is actually low and not simply a small notch down from intense. Some prefer even no power at all. That's where dildos come in. A dildo is an insertable toy that has no power of its own: you supply your own hand movement or thrusting power. You can combine a dildo with other toys, including ones that vibrate, for even more variation.

STYLE. What do you want to do with your toy? You might want a toy that's great for internal stimulation, in which case you'll want to be mindful of its length and width—according to your own preferences, of course. Then again, maybe you're seeking something non-penetrative that can spice up external vulva play—or even a multitasker that can offer internal and external pleasure all at once!

SHAPE. Maybe you want your toy to look like a penis, or a flower—or maybe you couldn't care less what the object looks like as long as it gets the job done. It's all good! Just be sure to choose a shape that appeals to you so that you like what you see when you're using it.

TEXTURE. Bumps on the surface of your toy will add a lot of extra stimulation, especially if you use it with lots of vigorous movement, which creates friction. Smoothly textured toys, on the other hand, glide over sensitive areas easily, but offer less intense sensation. Firm toys provide more pressure, which can be delicious (especially against the G-spot), while soft toys might be preferable when it comes to vigorous, deep thrusting (especially against the cervix).

SIZE. If you're looking for a toy you can insert vaginally, length and width can be an issue. If the toy is longer than your vagina, you'll have to hold yourself back to keep from inserting it all the way.

A toy that's too short can be equally frustrating, because it might not reach those specific pleasure spots, or it may keep popping out (to prevent this, choose a toy with a bulbous head). A toy that's too wide can be painful, while one that's too narrow can be unsatisfying. Even if you're only using it for external play, ask yourself whether you want a toy that feels hefty in your hand, or one that's petite and discreet? Think about what's worked well for you during your recent solo sex adventures, and choose one that'll be right for your needs.

MATERIAL. Because sex toys are an unregulated industry, you need to mind your own health by being a savvy shopper. Watch out for the disclaimer "For Novelty Purposes Only," which appears on the packaging for a lot of sex toys (especially the less-expensive ones). This means that the product is intended as a gag gift, so if you use it for sexual stimulation and end up with health problems as a result, the manufacturer won't be liable. This is an incredibly dishonest trick because, of course, it's obvious to everyone that such toys are in fact produced and marketed for sex play. So steer clear of toys that come with that disclaimer, and stick with ones that are made from these body-safe materials:

» SOFTER MATERIALS. Silicone and elastomer (TPR) are considered the safest options when it comes to softer toys. Be sure your silicone toys are made of 100 percent silicone: Many companies market their toys as silicone or "silicon," but some may contain as little as 10 percent of the desired material. Brands like LELO, JimmyJane, Vibratex, Fun Factory, Standard Innovation (We-vibe), Happy Valley/Fuze, Tantus, and Vixen all use the best-quality silicone. Latex toys are popular because they're softer and less expensive, but they often contain phthalates, which have been linked to fertility issues in some studies. They're also porous, which makes them harder to clean thoroughly. So, if you already have a favorite latex toy, play it safe by using a condom over it.

» FIRMER MATERIALS. Toys made from hard plastic, or plastic coated with a thin layer of silicone, are easy to find and safe to use. They provide satisfying pressure for the vulva, clitoris, and G-spot, and are good at conducting vibration throughout the length of the toy. Metal, glass, and wooden toys work well, too, and they do double duty as works of art! These body-safe, non-vibrating toys offer the weight and firm pressure that some women crave when it comes to more focused play, such as G-spot stimulation. (But they're not ideal for vigorous thrusting, which can be painful for your cervix.) Metal and glass are easy to sterilize in boiling water, so go ahead and share them safely with your new lover, a friend, or your sister! And they're pretty sturdy: Glass toys won't break unless you drop them from a height onto a hard surface. (If that happens, grip the toy with your hand and move your hand up and down, as if you were giving a hand job. If you can't feel any nicks or roughness, neither will your sensitive parts!) Wooden toys are tough, too, and as long as they're coated with a body-safe lacquer to prevent splintering, they're ready for pleasure.

QUALITY. Traditionally, sex toys were produced at about the same level of quality as dollar-store items. They weren't built to last, and most were knock-offs of higher-quality designs. This is still largely the case, unfortunately, but the good news is that these days, better-quality manufacturers are making top-notch toys with long lives: Some vibrators even come with ten-year warranties, while some dildos (without mechanical parts) sport lifetime warranties. You get what you pay for, so consider spending a few extra dollars for a trustworthy toy.

POWER SOURCE. Rechargeable or plug-in toys tend to be more expensive, but they last longer, and that means they're more eco-friendly (because fewer broken toys and batteries will end up in landfills). Plug-in toys offer less freedom to roam—but they won't die on you at inopportune moments (for example, just as you're about to come!). Battery-operated toys are often less expensive, but tend to be of poorer quality, and are more likely to break after several uses. If you do choose a battery-operated toy, try using rechargeable batteries with these toys, that way you get to love yourself and the planet at the same time.

THE "CADILLAC" OF VIBRATORS

You might have heard of the "Hitachi Magic Wand" massager, which appeared on the American market in the late 1960s. Produced as a back and muscle massager, it quickly became popular as an awesome vibrator, and it's gained international fame over the years. Recently, it's been rebranded as the "Original Magic Wand"—*sans* reference to Hitachi—but it's no less powerful than it ever was. It has two speeds: 5000 revolutions per minute (RPM) and 6000 RPM (translation: High and Really High). That means it can offer incredible intensity to those who need a little extra power to orgasm. And it's so powerful that its vibrations can penetrate to those deep erectile tissues that no weaker toy (or finger) could ever reach. Nicknamed the "Cadillac" of vibrators, it's loved by women because it's so reliable. It's a plug-in toy, so its power won't run out on you, and it lasts for years—even with daily use. Plus, its head has a large surface area. That means it covers a wide area of erectile tissue, not just a single spot on the clitoris. It can stimulate a lot of different sensitive spots at once, coaxing pleasure from a whole network of nerve endings.

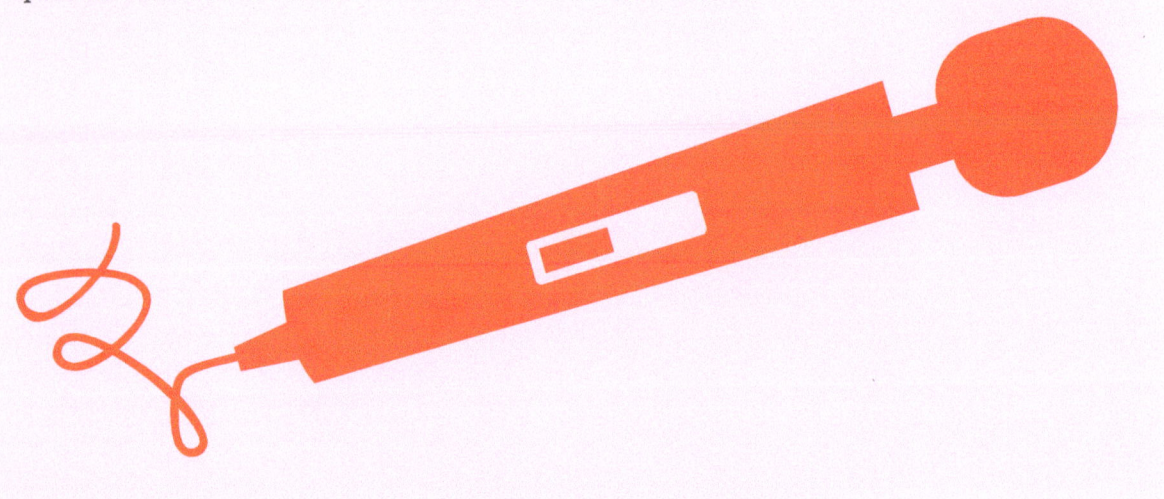

CAN I BECOME ADDICTED TO A VIBRATOR?

Don't worry: you can't get addicted to a vibrator—but you can become habituated to one. That's because everyone develops life habits that make getting through the day more efficient. The way you negotiate your commute to work or school (or anywhere else) is one such habit. If your car or bike breaks down, or if there's a transit strike and your usual train isn't running, you have to think a bit more and work a little harder at first as you figure out an alternative to your usual routine. If you usually drive, for example, you'll have to call someone to arrange a ride, or dust off your bike, or search your pockets for transit fare and a good book to read en route. But after a few days, you'll be used to your new routine, and you'll find you can easily switch back to it if you need to. Similarly, if you *always* masturbate in the *same* way with the *same* toy or technique, it might be hard to shift gears—at first. If you switch things up often—using your fingers instead of a toy, changing positions, or coming up with hot new fantasies—you'll be able to enjoy different kinds of pleasure quickly and easily.

According to Rachel P. Maines's book *The Technology of Orgasm: "Hysteria," the Vibrator, and Women's Sexual Satisfaction*, female hysteria (that is, expressing emotions) was considered a grave condition for which well-to-do women in the Victorian Era in Great Britain sought assistance from their medical doctors. Doctors believed hysteria to be caused by a woman's uterus floating around inside her body. Orgasm ("hysterical paroxysm") was the remedy to settle her uterus and thus her emotions. Her doctor would stimulate her clitoris with his hand until she climaxed. Despite the obvious popularity of this treatment, it was regarded as a medical procedure and not considered "sexual" due to the clinical context and the absence of any vaginal or penile involvement. Because the procedure of bringing their patients to orgasm with their hands was time-consuming and fatiguing, the vibrator was actually a medical invention designed to assist popular doctors in their orgasm-inducing work. Fortunately, the vibrator has come a long way since then!

VIBRATORS

You're ready to invest in a sex toy that's right for you—but where should you start? First, think about what you'd like to use your toy for. Are you dying to embark on a little G-spot exploration? Craving internal and external pleasure all at once? Want to hit your clit in the right spot? Here are a few suggestions to help guide you.

INTERNAL OR PENETRATIVE VIBRATORS
A GREAT ALL-ROUNDER:
Liv 2 vibrator by LELO: (www.lelo.com)

If you're looking to buy your first vibrator, the Liv 2 might be right for you. First-timers can use it to explore pleasure in all its forms: along the length of the vulva, on the clitoris, for general vaginal stimulation or G-spot pleasure, on the outside of the anus (this area is super-sensitive because it's full of nerve endings; just be sure to put a condom on your toy), or on the nipples. And just about any sex toy, including the Liv 2, can also be incorporated into partner sex (check out the "Toys for Two" sidebar on page 101 to find out how).

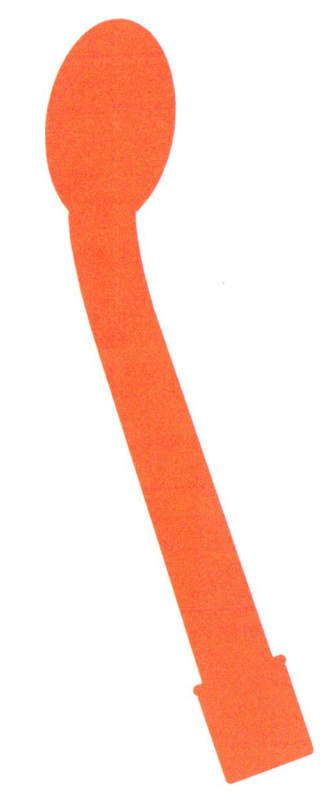

DETAILS: Firm silicone and acrylonitrile butadiene styrene (ABS) plastic toy. Rechargeable and waterproof, it comes with a 10-year warranty.

ALTERNATIVES: Any toy of your choice with the width and length that works for you.

AFFORDABLE G-SPOT DELIGHT:
Orchid Mood Frisky vibrator by Doc Johnson (www.docjohnson.com)

As versatile as the Liv 2, the Orchid is less expensive, and it's a great G-spot finder. The shaft is pretty long (and that's only a good thing!), but the most effective way to use it internally is to tilt it inside toward the belly button and pull the handle outward and downward against the opening of the vagina, rather than pushing it inside. The bulbous head will pull against the opening and front wall of the vagina, where most of the sensitive erectile tissues are.

DETAILS: This firm ABS plastic toy is water-resistant, takes two AA batteries, and does not include a warranty.

ALTERNATIVES: Any toy of your choice with a bulbous head and/or a curve.

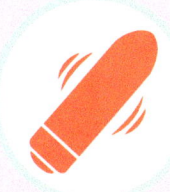

TOYS FOR TWO

Bringing a sex toy into the bedroom? Don't hog all the fun for yourself! With just a little creativity, you can use sex toys to pump up the pleasure for both you and your partner. If your partner's a woman, use your favorite toy techniques on her, and see how she responds. Or try placing the toy between you so that you can both grind against it. If your partner has a penis, roll the toy around his shaft, or cup his testicles and gently stimulate them with it. Then, place the broadest side of the toy against his perineum (or "manbridge"). The base of his penis is buried deep below the perineum, so the vibrations will rock his world. You can also use toys to spice up oral sex, whether your partner's male or female: just hold the toy against your cheek to give your partner a wild ride as you're going down. Stimulate your partner's nipples with your vibe (and take note: many men need regular nipple stimulation before they notice how good it feels!). And, of course, simply place your toy against your clitoris during intercourse, or use it during partner sex in the same way you would if you were flying solo.

· · · · · · · · · · ·

THRUSTER: Stronic Zwei Pulsator by Fun Factory (www.funfactory.com)

Most vibrators vibrate (well, obviously!), but few of them actually thrust in and out. Enter the Stronic: If you like fast, short movements either externally or internally, this toy has your number. But of course you may like the thrusting sensation also on the outside, to rub your vulva and/or clitoris without moving your hand. Also great for the G-spot and can be used anally for anyone who can accommodate a bit of girth in the butt.

DETAILS: This soft silicone toy is waterproof and rechargeable, and comes with a 2-year warranty.

ALTERNATIVES: None! This vibrator's truly unique: it's the only one of its kind.

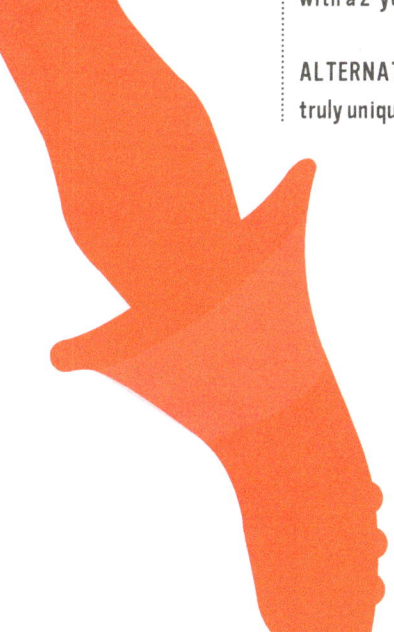

THE INFAMOUS RABBIT EARS:
Vanity Rabbit by Jopen
(www.jopenvibrators.com)

Made famous by *Sex and the City*, the rabbit vibrator is so fabulous that it's inspired countless knock-offs, which are generally inferior in terms of quality. Not the Vanity Rabbit, though! This top-quality toy provides hours of pleasure that, according to some women, feels like oral sex. That's due to its rotating shaft, which enables the rabbit ears to dance around the clitoris. Some women love it because it offers satisfying G-spot pleasure, but for others, the feeling of "fullness" during penetration combined with the unparalleled sensations of the rabbit ears really nudges them over the edge. The ears can also be used on their own—on the clitoris, anus, frenulum (underside of the penis's head), or nipples.

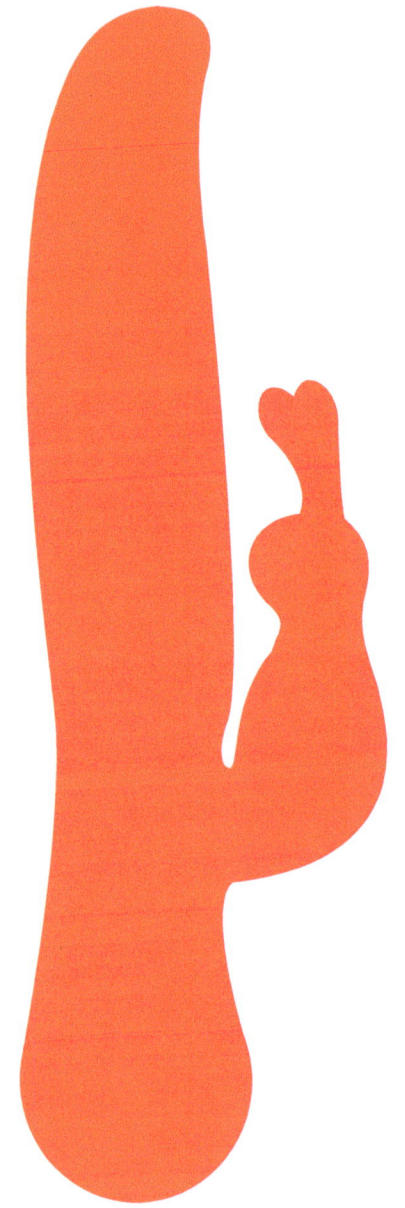

DETAILS: This soft silicone toy is rechargeable and waterproof, and comes with a 2-year warranty.

ALTERNATIVES: It's hard to beat the Vanity Rabbit, because many knock-offs don't have rotating shafts. And other animal-themed vibrators—like dolphins or beavers—lack one major advantage: the two "ticklers" that provide more indirect stimulation to both sides of the clitoris. (Some women find that the direct pressure of one tickler can be too intense for the clit.) That said, some alternative toys feature sacs of rotating beads at the base of the shaft, and they do feel pleasurable when they're pressed up against the sensitive opening of the vagina.

ALL-AT-ONCE: Ina 2 vibrator by LELO (www.lelo.com)

Lusting after internal and external pleasure at the same time? Grab the Ina 2. It's got different functions and pulses, and it has two motors, so you can use them together—for an especially sumptuous sensation—or one at a time. It's also great for external use only: place one part against the clitoris and the other against the opening to the vagina.

DETAILS: This firm silicone toy is rechargeable and waterproof, and comes with a 10-year warranty.

ALTERNATIVES: Some knock-offs of the Ina 2 don't deliver, so if you decide to purchase a similar toy, make sure that the clitoral branch of your toy is actually long enough to reach your clitoris!

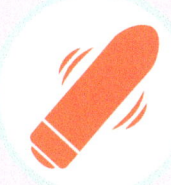

CHANGE MEANS PLEASURE

When you find that special spot with your vibrator, it's so tempting to stay there; after all, if it feels good, why put it anywhere else? Well, here's why: Repetition can numb your senses. For instance, if a friend or partner rubs your arm in the same way for more than a minute, the amazing sensation you felt at first quickly fades into the background. Or if you walk out into a noisy street after chatting with a friend in a quiet café, you'll notice the contrast in environments first, but your brain will soon adjust to the new level of background sound. Your body perceives and rewards difference, so when a sound or sensation remains the same for a while, your body will ignore that stimulus so it can focus on new ones. And as with life, so with vibrators. If you leave your vibrator in one spot for long, your nerve endings will stop responding. But as long as you continue to move it—even slightly—your body will stay sensitive to pleasure. Plus, rhythmic back-and-forth, up-and-down, or in-and-out motions are helpful when it comes to achieving orgasm. So when you find that sweet spot, stay there, but be sure to move your toy in the rhythm that feels right to you. That way, you'll keep up the intensity—and the pleasure.

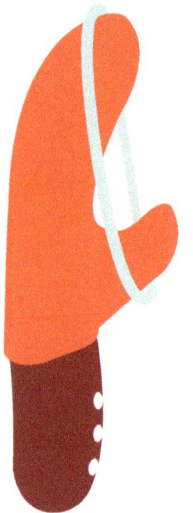

SMALLER AND FULLER: The Amorino by Fun Factory (www.funfactory.com)

If you're after a smaller-sized toy that's great for internal and external play, try the Amorino. Its best feature is its removable stimulation band, a length of stretchy silicone that conducts the toy's vibrations through the labia. The result? Amazing pleasure for the vulva, alongside satisfying clitoral and vaginal stimulation.

DETAILS: This soft silicone toy is rechargeable and waterproof, and comes with a 2-year warranty.

ALTERNATIVES: Any toy that is smaller with two branches, but it will be hard to find a different one with the unique silicone elastic band!

SOMETHING COMPLETELY DIFFERENT: We-Vibe 4 Plus by We-Vibe (www.we-vibe.com)

This remote-controlled toy has a fabulous reputation, especially for use during intercourse (vibration for the clitoris and for the G-spot *plus* penis- or dildo-thrusting equals *wow*!). But it's also amazing for solo play. The We-Vibe 4 Plus is pretty small in size, but it offers medium-intensity stimulation both internally and externally. If you dare, try wearing it under your clothes to your next boring work meeting, gym workout, or pub night. Because you control the vibrations with the remote, no one will know that you're in the throes of pleasure—unless you start moaning, that is. Or your partner can control the vibrations from the same room or through his or her smartphone from across the world. Alternatively, like most sex toys, it can be used both vaginally and anally (be sure to put a condom over it first), or you can wear it under a strap-on dildo to buzz yourself while penetrating a partner.

DETAILS: This firm but flexible silicone toy is rechargeable and waterproof, and comes with a 1-year warranty.

ALTERNATIVES: Toys with a larger internal piece can give you more of a sense of fullness, but they're a bit more challenging to also use during penetration with a toy or penis. Some alternative options also have a vibrating remote, which gives you the chance to double your pleasure!

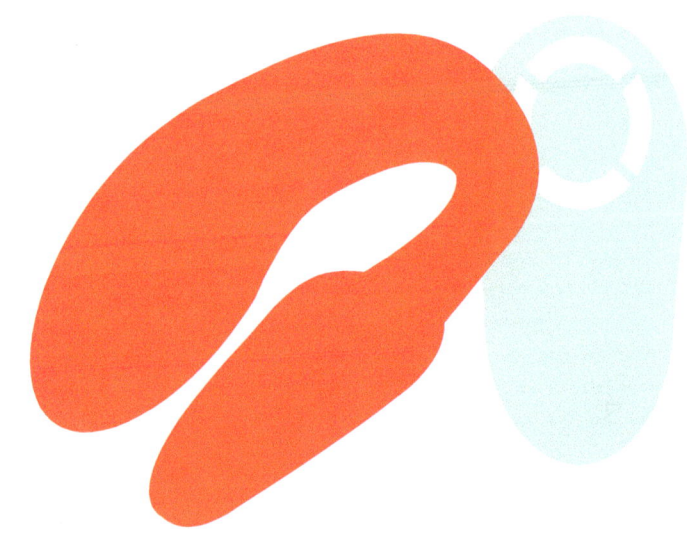

SOFT AND SERIOUS: The Tiger by Fun Factory (www.funfactory.com)

The Tiger is a soft toy that's perfect for full, deep stimulation. It has a small bump on the outside that may hit your clitoris, so it might be able to do double duty—but that's not how it earned its reputation. It's so popular because it delivers nearly the same sensation as intercourse does. You can also use it solo or partnered along the vulva, the clitoris, for general vaginal stimulation, on the outside of the anus, or on the nipples.

DETAILS: This soft, flexible silicone toy is rechargeable and waterproof, and comes with a 2-year warranty.

ALTERNATIVES: Other soft toys with cushiony heads in whichever size and shape works for you.

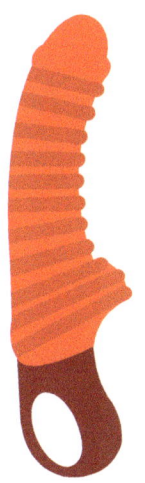

TWO-PRONGED APPROACH: Leaf Vitality by BMS Enterprises (www.bmsfactory.com)

Like the We-Vibe or Ina 2, the Leaf Vitality can be used internally and externally. It has two curved ends that resemble sprouting leaves or branches, and both ends can be used for either kind of play. Spreading the branches apart and pressing down on the base will push one end up toward the clitoris and the other toward the anus, which makes for satisfying external stimulation. You can also insert one branch into the vagina, leaving the other side free to pleasure the clitoris, vulva, or anus. Or place a condom over one end, and insert it into your anus, and let the other end rub against your vulva. Slide both branches into the vagina so that one branch stimulates the front wall of the vagina (G-spot alert!) while the other pleasures the perineal sponge that's located at the back wall of the vagina. Or squeeze the two branches together around the nipples or the underside of the penis.

DETAILS: This firm but pliable silicone toy is rechargeable and waterproof, and comes with a 10-year warranty.

ALTERNATIVES: Any toy that offers two flexible silicone branches.

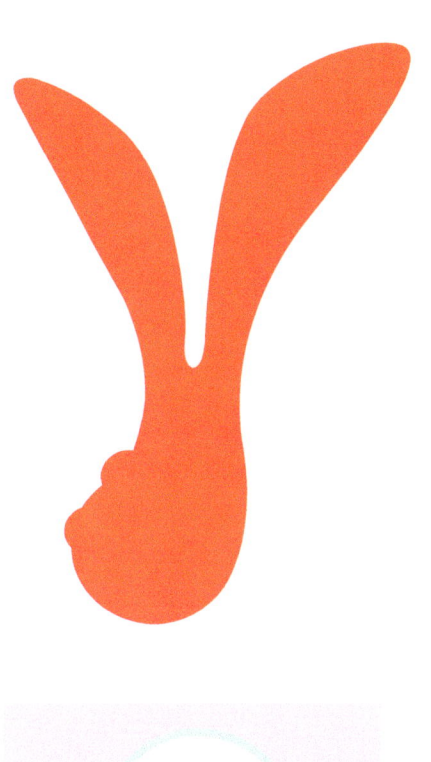

A MATCH MADE IN HEAVEN

Eight out of ten women who use vibrators generally use the pressure of the vibrator directly against the clitoris.

EXTERNAL OR NON-PENETRATIVE VIBRATORS

THE TOOTH: Form 2 vibrator by JimmyJane (www.jimmyjane.com)

Sound scary? It's not! The Form 2 is shaped like an upside-down tooth, which means it has two (very, very versatile) prongs. You can use them to stimulate either or both sides of the clitoris; you can run them up and down your labia; or you can tease your nipples with them. Alternatively, hold on to the prongs and use the flatter end of the toy on your vulva, or against your partner's testicles, perineum, or anus. The Form 2 packs powerful vibrations and vibration modes into a toy that's smaller than your hand, making it an incredibly exciting tool for external play.

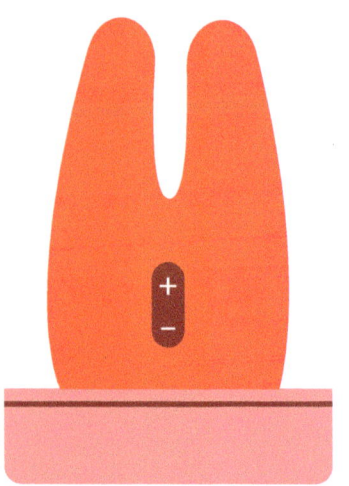

DETAILS: This firm but pliable silicone toy is rechargeable and waterproof, and comes with a 3-year warranty.

ALTERNATIVES: Any toy with two branches or prongs that are close to one another can be used in the same way.

STYLISH DISGUISE: Mia 2 Vibrator by LELO (www.lelo.com)

If spontaneity's your thing, you won't be able to live without the Mia 2. No bigger than a lipstick, it can be popped into your purse and taken with you just about anywhere. What's more, it recharges via USB connection, so if you're traveling with your laptop, you'll have an instant power source. (Not that you'll need to recharge it that often, because it lasts for an hour and a half after it's fully charged.) You can use it solo or partnered along the vulva, the clitoris, on the outside of the anus, or on the nipples. Like most toys, it's great for partnered play, too: check out the "Toys for Two" sidebar on page 101 to find out how to make the Mia 2 work for both of you.

DETAILS: Made of firm ABS plastic, this toy is waterproof and rechargeable, and comes with a 10-year warranty.

ALTERNATIVES: Anything small and powerful! Do your research first, though: Most toys that are designed to look like lipstick or other cosmetics may be cute, but they're generally poor quality.

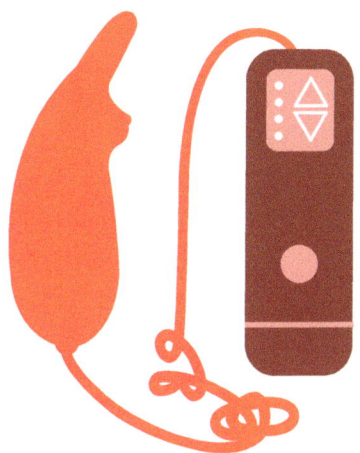

THE EGG WITH BENEFITS: Mardi Gras Rabbit (www.gtadulttoys.com)

This fabulous toy packs all the pleasure of both an egg and a rabbit-style vibrator into a miniature version that's less expensive, too. Its shape makes it so versatile, so you can mix and match the three different sensations the toy offers: the tickliness of the rabbit's ears, the soft squishiness of its nose, and the firm pressure of the egg-shaped base.

DETAILS: Made of thermoplastic elastomer, this soft toy is waterproof, takes two AA batteries, and does not include a warranty.

ALTERNATIVES: Any egg-style toy is a great starter option if you're a first-timer; some even come with rabbit-style attachments.

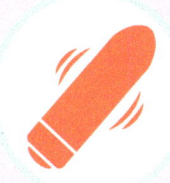

VIBRATORS AND DILDOS: WHAT'S THE DIFFERENCE?

A vibrator has a power source. It might use batteries, or it might be rechargeable, like a cell phone, or it might plug directly into a wall socket. Your vibrator will have buttons that turn it on and off, and to change the speed and intensity of the vibration. A dildo, on the other hand, has no power: you have to supply your own.

That might sound like more work, but it's totally worth it. You can squeeze, press, thrust, or slide a dildo inside you, or you can even put a vibrator against a dildo to make it vibrate once it's inside. They definitely have their advantages!

OTHER

ANAL BEGINNER: Quattro Butt Plug by FuzeToys (www.fuzetoys.com)

This simple, narrow toy can help you explore anal pleasure for the first time. Insert it, then leave it in place while you play with other erogenous zones, or use plenty of lube and slowly move it in and out: it's got four lobes that make penetration extra pleasurable. Its vibrator is removable, which means you can easily sterilize the Quattro by boiling it. (Non-creamy soap or toy cleaner plus water will also do the trick if you're only using it on yourself.)

DETAILS: This soft silicone toy is waterproof and uses watch batteries. The silicone toy (minus the removable vibe) comes with a lifetime warranty.

ALTERNATIVES: Experiment with anal toys of different lengths, widths, and styles of vibration.

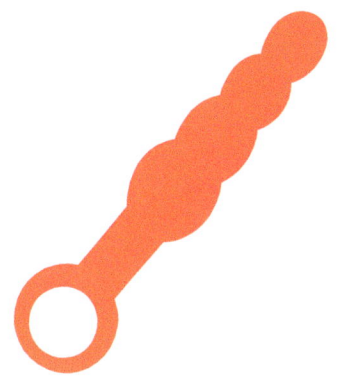

NON-VIBRATING TOYS

Pleasure doesn't have to vibrate. There are plenty of other sex toys that'll keep you amused during your next solo sex romp!

PURE WAND BY NJOY: If you're not into vibration, grab the Pure Wand: I all but guarantee that it'll help you find your G-spot. It's made from stainless steel, and the weight and pressure of the metal feel amazing, so use either the smaller or larger end, and curve it up inside you. Pull it out against your vaginal opening for added delight. (Bonus: It also has a great reputation for prostate pleasure for men.) (www.njoytoys.com)

SILICONE DILDO: If you love the "full" feeling of a toy or penis inside your vagina, try a pure silicone toy dildo. Dildos produced by Tantus (www.tantusinc.com) and Happy Valley (www.happyvalleysilicone.com) sport a good balance between firmness of pressure, ripples (for G-spot stimulation), and comfortable softness. Or if you're after something even softer that looks and feels realistic, try VixSkin toys (www.vixencreations .com); they have super-soft cushiony heads, and are just the thing for deeper, more intense thrusting.

NIPPLE CLAMPS: Like having your nipples squeezed, but just haven't got enough hands to do it all at the same time? Nipple clamps are your answer! They're adjustable, so you can play from mild to wild and anywhere in between. Here's a handy rule of thumb: The thinner the clamp, the more "pinchy" the sensation will be, while a broader clamp will deliver more pressure than pinch. And tips with rounded edges tend to be a better fit for women's nipples.

LUNA BEADS BY LELO: You already know that strengthening your PC or pelvic floor muscles will improve your orgasms. So grab a "string" of Luna beads, and get your squeeze on! Luna beads are small balls that you can insert one or two at a time, and each bead consists of a smaller ball inside a slightly larger outer ball. The inner ball rolls around inside the outer one whenever you move, giving you a secret hit of pleasure, and reminding you to do your pelvic floor squeezes. And doing them will feel great, because the inner part of the clitoris is sandwiched between the PC muscles. What all this means is you can have sex *and* exercise while you're shopping, walking the dog, or vacuuming! (There are plenty of alternatives to this toy, but most don't feature an inner ball inside an outer ball, which is such a huge part of what makes it so fun.) (www.lelo.com)

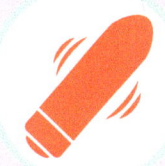

DON'T FORGET THE LUBE!

This is probably old news to you now, because you've read all about it in chapter 4, but lube is important for sexual pleasure. Whether you're using toys, fingers, or other objects that look like fun, everything feels way better with lube. It reduces friction, and just helps everything glide easily. Even if your body produces lots of natural lubrication when you're having sex, you may still need a little extra help, especially if you're using toys externally. So lube up before you start playing with any of the toys featured in this chapter.

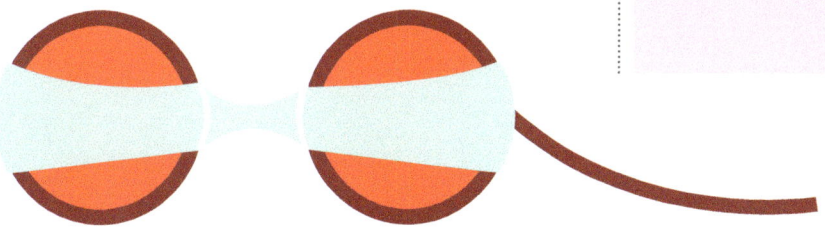

HOW TO CHOOSE A VIBRATOR

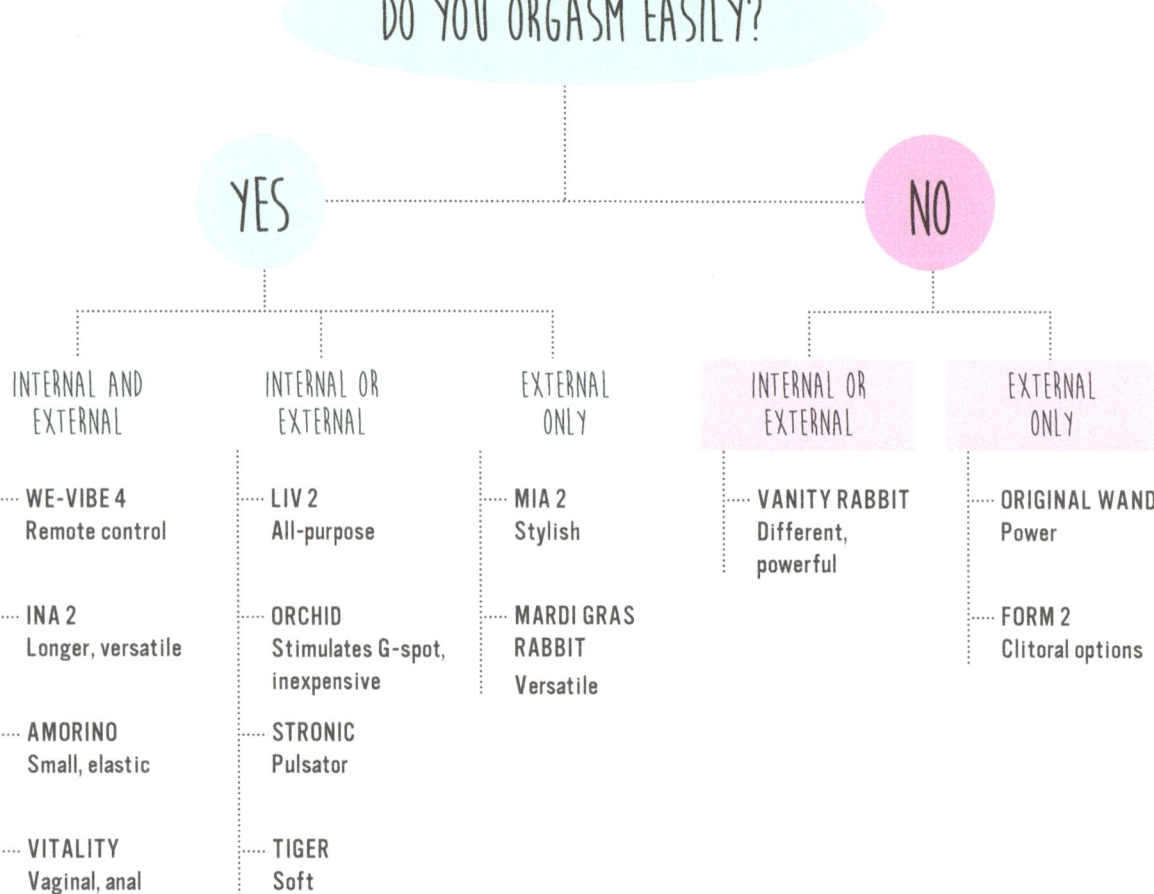

DO YOU ORGASM EASILY?

YES

INTERNAL AND EXTERNAL

- **WE-VIBE 4**
  Remote control

- **INA 2**
  Longer, versatile

- **AMORINO**
  Small, elastic

- **VITALITY**
  Vaginal, anal

INTERNAL OR EXTERNAL

- **LIV 2**
  All-purpose

- **ORCHID**
  Stimulates G-spot, inexpensive

- **STRONIC**
  Pulsator

- **TIGER**
  Soft

EXTERNAL ONLY

- **MIA 2**
  Stylish

- **MARDI GRAS RABBIT**
  Versatile

NO

INTERNAL OR EXTERNAL

- **VANITY RABBIT**
  Different, powerful

EXTERNAL ONLY

- **ORIGINAL WAND**
  Power

- **FORM 2**
  Clitoral options

HOW TO CLEAN YOUR TOYS

When you were a kid, you were probably told to put away your toys when you were finished playing with them. Same goes for sex toys, but there's an extra step involved: It's important to clean them thoroughly before putting them away. Soap and water are all you need, but be mindful of your soap's ingredients. Lots of soaps are fortified with a creamy oil that's meant to soften your hands, but it can damage latex and silicone toys. Stick with clear glycerin soap or a toy cleaner. Beware of those that contain parabens, which may be carcinogenic, or nonoxynol-9, an abrasively powerful cleansing agent that's used as a spermicide. Instead, go for a natural product like Diva Wash, which is safe for after-play cleanup. (Diva Wash is also safe for washing your vulva. Although it's not necessary to use soap, if you do choose to wash your vulva, you'll want a pH-balanced product that'll maintain your body's natural ecology. And remember that you don't need to put anything inside your vagina to clean it: doing so gets rid of your body's "good" bacteria and can even cause yeast infections.) Once your toys are clean, store them in a lint-free bag or a clean box, and keep them in an easy-to-find place. You don't want to be scouring your cupboards and shelves looking for your favorite supplies when the urge for pleasure strikes!

Sex, in all its forms, is about exploration and experimentation, and playing with sex toys is a great way to do just that. Pay attention to how you feel as you go: if one toy is too small, you've learned you'll need a bigger one next time (and you can save the smaller one for anal pleasure). If your toy is too hard, invest in a softer one, or try using it when you're more aroused. If your lubricant dries out too quickly, find a longer lasting one. There's always more to learn, and that's the beauty of solo sex. So keep reading: Chapter 6 will show you how to keep sex with yourself hot, year after year.

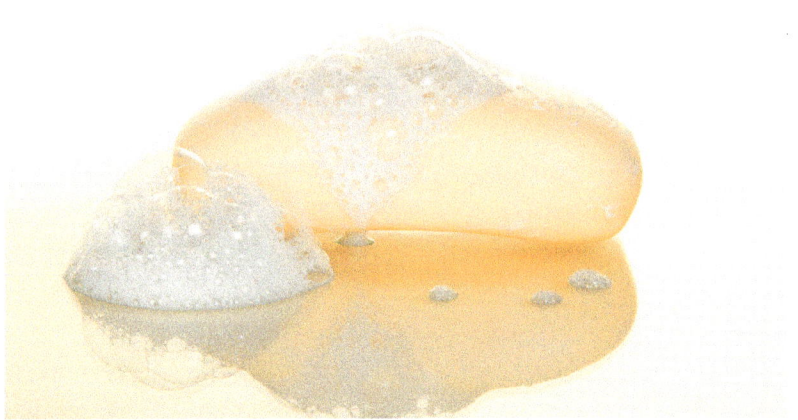

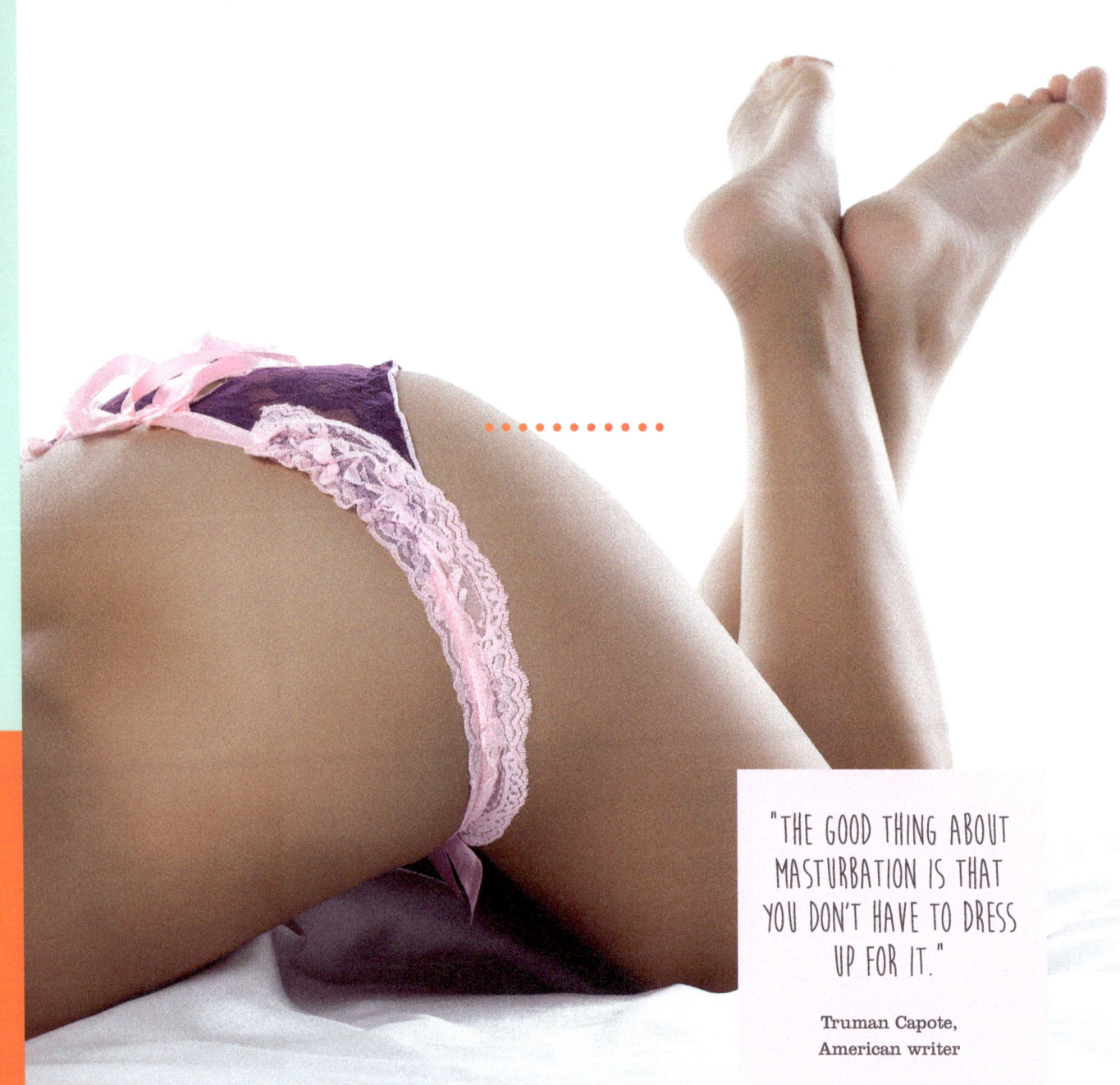

"THE GOOD THING ABOUT MASTURBATION IS THAT YOU DON'T HAVE TO DRESS UP FOR IT."

Truman Capote,
American writer

SPICING IT UP:

6

KEEP YOUR SOLO SEX ROUTINE FUN, HOT, AND EXCITING

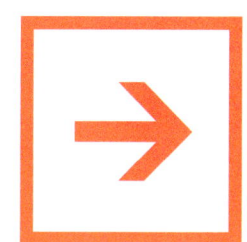

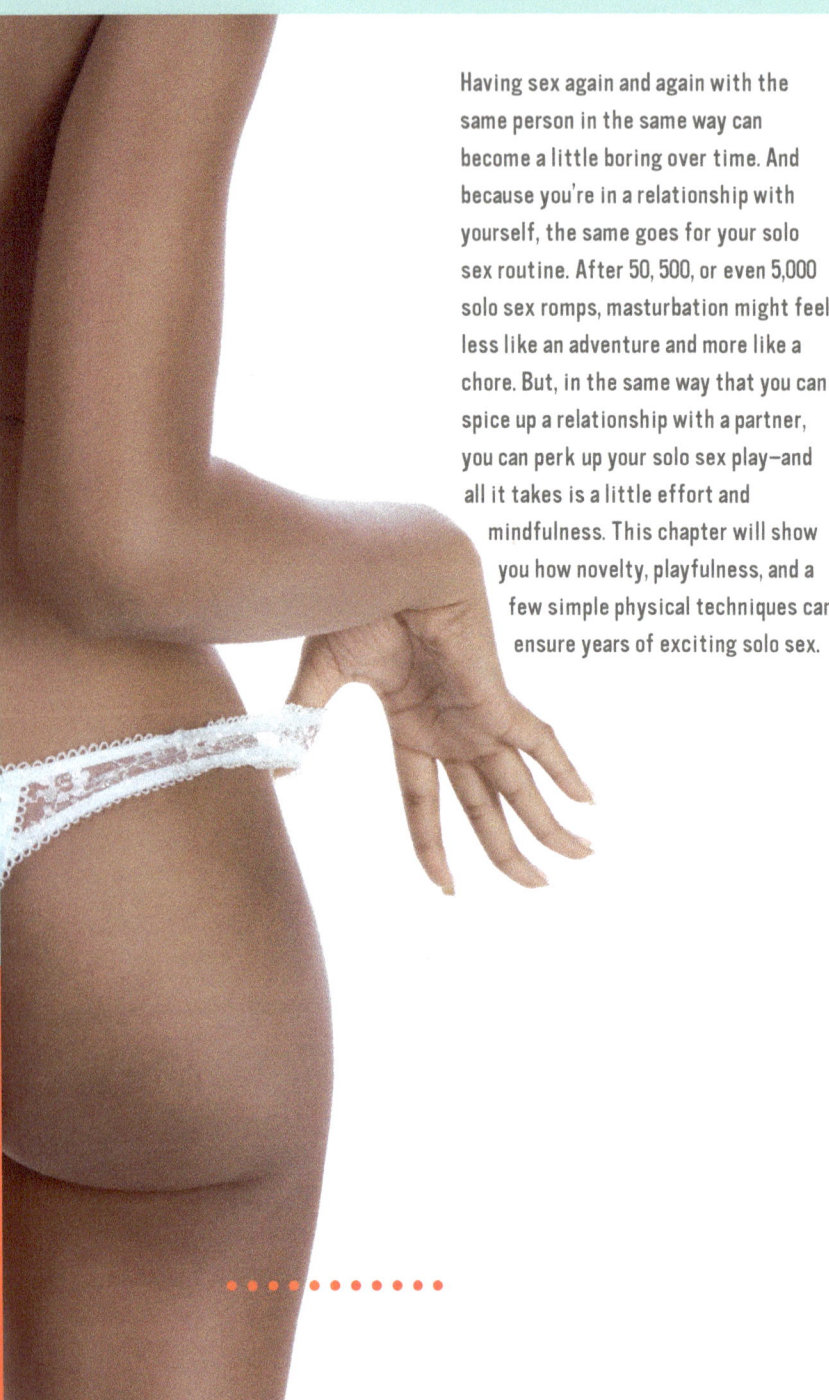

Having sex again and again with the same person in the same way can become a little boring over time. And because you're in a relationship with yourself, the same goes for your solo sex routine. After 50, 500, or even 5,000 solo sex romps, masturbation might feel less like an adventure and more like a chore. But, in the same way that you can spice up a relationship with a partner, you can perk up your solo sex play—and all it takes is a little effort and mindfulness. This chapter will show you how novelty, playfulness, and a few simple physical techniques can ensure years of exciting solo sex.

EMBRACE PLAY

As you discovered in chapter 3, your body responds better to pleasure once you're relaxed. There's no doubt about it: Relaxing helps you experience arousal and pleasure to its fullest extent. Can there be too much of a good thing, though? Definitely. Being *too* relaxed during solo sex might make you feel sleepy, or just plain old bored. That's why adding a little "edge" or risk to solo sex sessions can boost your arousal in a big way. For example—if it turns you on— the possibility of being caught in the act can make pleasure that much more intense. Or if that's not up your alley, you could try a new toy, new location, new technique, new position, new type of stimulation, new taboo, new goal, or new fantasy. You could play as usual, using your nondominant hand for a change, or without a technique or toy you generally rely on. What about playing a game with yourself? How many orgasms can you have within, say, half an hour, or however long a solo sex session takes? How long can you delay orgasm before you just have to let go? Make friends with your inner child—she loves turning tasks into games. And there are countless ways to play!

Masturbation offers the perfect opportunity to expand your fantasy life. Because you don't have to be concerned about what a partner would think, want, or do, your imagination can run wild—and it can lead you into uncharted, taboo, or unrealistic territory. And that's a great thing! You could imagine having sex with your boss, your ex, your friend's partner, or your favorite porn star, Hollywood star, or musician. You can try on any number of roles or power relationships for size: think teacher-and-student, doctor-and-patient, boss-and-assistant, firefighter-and-victim, or masseur-and-client. Using nothing but your imagination, you can play out scenes you might never encounter (or even want) in real life, like anal sex, strap-on sex, domination, or submission. And you can fantasize about sex on Mars, in your parents' bedroom, on your boss's desk, or on a park bench. The fantasy world is absolutely limitless, and incredibly exciting. If it feels right to you, think about sharing your fantasies with your partner. They might be trial runs for situations you'd like to experience in real life—or not. Lots of fantasies are best left as just that: fantasies.

I FANTASIZE ABOUT BEING RAPED. IS THAT OKAY?

Having rape fantasies makes lots of people, especially women, feel uncomfortable. That's understandable: It's unlikely that anyone would want that to happen in real life, so why fantasize about it? First of all, know that you are not alone. Between 31 percent and 57 percent of women have fantasies that involve sex against their will. Secondly, having rape fantasies doesn't necessarily mean that you were sexually abused, or that you want to be. Rape fantasies usually occur in a very controlled way: Most of the time, they involve someone *you* choose whom *you* find attractive, who is approaching you in a way that *you* find erotic, and who is having his or her way with you in a manner that *you* secretly enjoy. The fact is, actual rape doesn't contain *any* of those controlled elements. What's more, such fantasies are often about a pleasurable loss of control, in which you're so irresistible to your fantasy lover that they just can't keep their hands off of you. It's about being desired and experiencing excitement and pleasure while surrendering control. Yes, control is surrendered in rape fantasies, but, as in any fantasy, it's enacted in ways that you enjoy.

LOCATION, LOCATION, LOCATION

Fantasizing about having sex in different places is great, but the best part is, you can actually have solo sex in some of those places! Okay, so masturbating in a back alley probably isn't the best idea, but there are still lots of semi-public places where you can enjoy some hot solo sex. Bear in mind that masturbating in public is illegal. Plus, as in all forms of sex, consent is important: It's true that the person who accidentally discovers you getting busy in that back alley while walking her dog might find it exciting, but it's more likely that she'll feel offended or violated. (Masturbating in public can be dangerous for you, too.) So get creative, and try playing in a few new locations: in different parts of your house or apartment, in a sex club (if that turns you on), or in a very secluded part of the great outdoors (preferably on your own property).

Whether you're fantasizing about solo sex in an exciting location or are actually there, go ahead and play with different positions. If you're imagining yourself in an especially exciting sex position, get into it! That'll make the fantasy seem more realistic, and you might discover a new way to masturbate to boot. Here are a few suggestions: Try lying on your tummy and grinding against your hand or a toy. Lie on your back and bring your knees to your chest in a fetal position, then reach around from behind your thighs. Get on all fours as though you were having sex "on top" and crouch over a toy that's nestled in a pillow, suctioned to a wall, or attached to a chair. Or just kneel and play as you look out the window, watch some porn, or watch yourself in the mirror. (In this position, it often helps to have something to brace yourself against, such as a wall, backboard, chair, or sofa.) Lie on your side with feet outstretched, in a fetal position, or with each leg in a different position. Go at it standing up—then try to not fall when orgasmic bliss hits. Park yourself on the bed, chair, couch, stairs, desk, or kitchen counter; sit in the tub, on the toilet, or on the clothes dryer. Each new position can be a fun challenge!

Try varying the times of day at which you enjoy solo sex. If you usually do it before bed, try it in the mornings, right after waking up, or as an afternoon delight, or as a cocktail before going out on a date in the evening. Your energy and arousal will vary at different times of day, and so will your solo sex play.

TABOOS

Taboos can be fodder for amazing erotic fantasies. Anything you consider "forbidden" is bound to be more exciting—even before your solo sex session kicks off! Think about this: what are your personal taboos? (Each person's response will be different.) Is it oral sex—giving, receiving, or swallowing? Maybe it's anal play, kink, surrendering your power to someone else, having an adventure with a person of a particular gender, dressing up as someone of a different gender, dirty talk, strap-on play, being watched, group sex, paying for sex, or being paid for sex. The list goes on and on! Again, some of these taboo scenes may not be possible, plausible, or realistic, while others can be acted out in real life. Either way, use props such as clothing, toys, and accessories (plus your imagination, of course!) to enhance the experience and make it as realistic as you can. Nothing's forbidden in the world of fantasy.

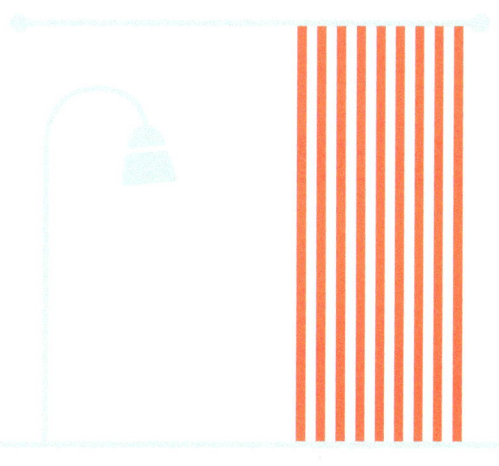

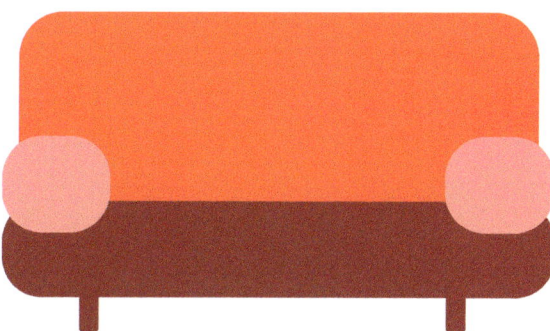

CREATE AN AMBIENCE

You already know that setting the mood can take partner sex from so-so to so hot. Same goes for solo sex. Try to incorporate as many of your senses as possible, because each detail contributes to a heightened experience, but the setup doesn't have to be complicated or time-consuming.

» TOUCH. Pay attention to your entire body. Start by applying your favorite lotion or body oil, or get into a hot bath and use textured soap to caress your body from head to foot. Run Mardi Gras beads or other textured objects along the length of your body (see chapter 5 for a few ideas). All of these things will help you relax, stay in the present moment, and get into the mood—and they turn pleasure into a full-body experience.

» SOUND. Choose a few tunes based on the atmosphere you want to create, whether it's upbeat, relaxing, sensual, sexy, or arousing. Turning on the music can also help drown out any noises that aren't terribly sexy, like the TV in the next room, the construction going on next door, or the kids playing outside. (Plus, it's helpful if other people are nearby as it camouflages any pleasurable sounds you might make during solo sex.) Speaking of volume level, if your vibrator makes a lot of noise when it's on, you might worry that the entire block will know when you're masturbating! Here's how to ease your mind: turn on your toy, and put it on your bed (or wherever else you plan on using it). Close the door to the room, and wander around your home. If you can't hear it in the next room, know that no one else will, either.

» VISUAL. Fire up the candles, dim the lights, or go to your favorite outdoor secluded location, because visuals can be a major part of solo sex sessions. (So can the lack of visuals: Blindfolding yourself will heighten all your other senses!) Think about watching yourself masturbate in the mirror, or turn on a sexy movie. Some Hollywood scenes that are masturbation-worthy include those from *9 1/2 Weeks*, *Basic Instinct*, *Bound*, *Out of Africa*, and *The Notebook*—or just about anything that features your favorite actor. Or you could try an erotic film; if you're not impressed with or aroused by most mainstream offerings, know that there are plenty of women-friendly alternatives. For heterosexual preferences, try flicks produced by Lust Films, Ovidie, Sweet Sensations or Joybear. For lesbian, bi, or queer sensibilities (which many women of all orientations can enjoy), try Trouble Films, Pink and White, Triangle Films, or Philly Films.

» SMELL. Pop a few drops of your favorite essential oil into your bath or diffuser, and breathe deeply. Light a scented candle; drape an object made of leather, such as a coat, skirt, or belt, over your face; or place some scented flowers on your bedside table. Smell is a powerful, visceral sense that can stir your blood in ways that your other senses can't. So go ahead and indulge yourself!

» TASTE. Eating during sex is probably a little too challenging to manage, but you can easily suck on a decadent chocolate, a jellybean, or a lollipop (lollipops are great, because the stick will prevent choking). Luscious flavors can round out the experience, and a particular flavor can help evoke a fantasy, or transport you back to an especially sexy time or place.

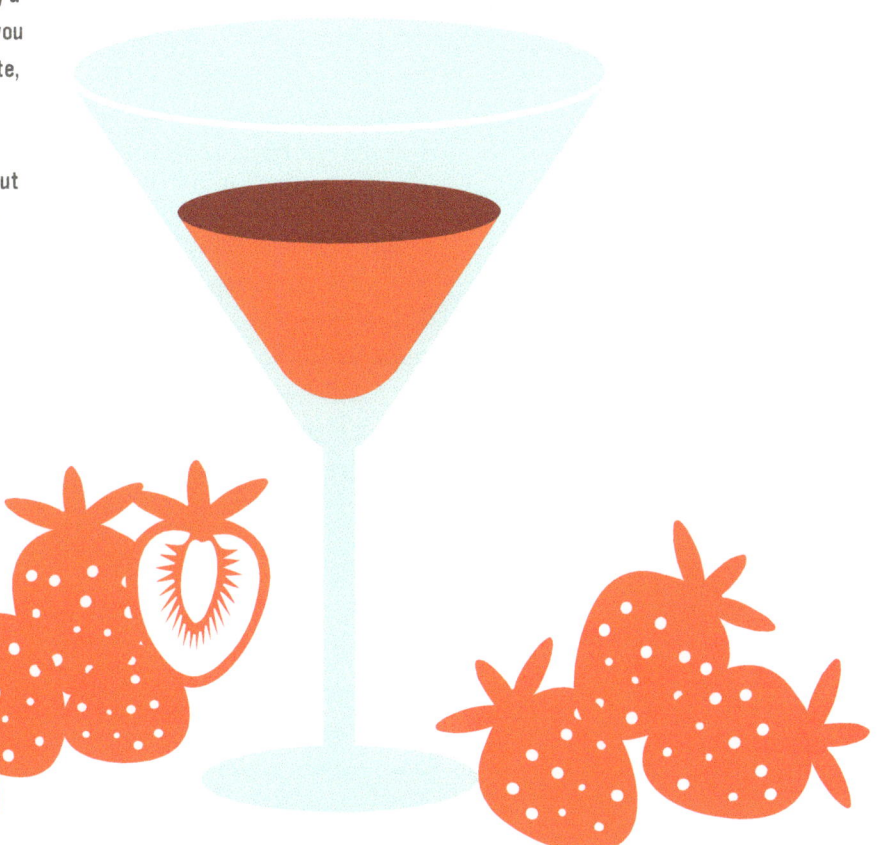

PHYSICAL TECHNIQUES FOR EXTRA PLEASURE

Being open-minded and playful, creating a relaxing, sensuous ambience, and tapping into taboo subjects can all help get you in the mood, but a few simple physical techniques can ramp up your solo sex play, too. Of course, these techniques work whether you're flying solo or as a duo, but practicing them solo means you get to learn and experiment without feeling self-conscious—and that makes it easier to reinforce your new habits. Like any skill, the more you practice new solo sex habits, the less you'll have to think about them, and the more natural they'll become. Eventually, you'll feel like you've been doing them forever! So, take note of these eight tips.

» BE SURE TO BREATHE. Because you're alive, you're already breathing, but breathing deeply and fully actually helps you experience pleasure more intensely. Breath carries both intention and blood to our genitals, essential ingredients for sex of any kind! Lots of people breathe shallowly and quickly, especially when aroused: that's natural, but breathing more fully helps oxygen circulate throughout your bloodstream, and fills you with even more erotic energy. So be mindful of your breath during solo sex.

» MAKE SOME SOUNDS. Maybe you're already a vigorous screamer. If that's the case, muffle your screams with a pillow, or challenge yourself to be as quiet as you can—it'll add a whole new dimension of eroticism to your solo play. But if you're like most people, you might be too shy to make noise, or maybe you've had to practice having sex quietly for so many years that it's become second nature. If so, add some sound effects to your sex sessions. In the same way that athletes often make sounds to help them focus on their physical movements— think of the way tennis players grunt as they hit the ball—you can boost your pleasure levels by making sounds that feel natural to you. Don't worry: You don't have to go all-out and pretend to be a porn star (but go for it if that turns you on!). Just allow yourself to sigh as you breathe out: it might sound like a lazy "ahhhhh." Simply let the sound fall out of your mouth. No one is around to judge you, so don't be shy. Remember that it's not about how loud you are; you won't get extra points for screaming. Instead, it's about how authentic your expression of pleasure is. How does this help your solo sex sessions in general? Well, if you're suppressing one way in which your body usually expresses pleasure—via your voice—then you're probably holding your body back from expressing pleasure in other ways, too. Instead, let your voice express and enhance your arousal.

» DO PELVIC FLOOR SQUEEZES. You know pelvic floor squeezes are important for your health, but did you know that strong PC muscles can also intensify sexual pleasure and orgasm? Try them during solo or partner sex; it'll feel fabulous, because your clitoris is sandwiched right between those muscles. It's also a great way to get over the "hump" when you're close to orgasm: a few well-timed squeezes can push you right over the edge. And, of course, you can also do pelvic floor exercises when you're not having sex. Either way, they'll strengthen your PC muscles, which means you'll have better orgasms and fewer health problems. People with weak pelvic floor muscles tend to experience incontinence, or in more serious cases, prolapse of the bladder through the wall of the vagina. That can be incredibly painful and can even require surgery. So keep squeezing!

» MOVE YOUR PELVIS. This one's best done in private! Gently rocking your pelvis will enhance your pleasure when you're getting it on alone. Rocking your pelvis keeps it "open," so to speak, so that the nerves that pass through your sacrum can keep the pleasure flowing without hindrance. Simply moving your pelvis gently or rocking it back and forth will do the trick.

SEX IN SECRET?

Want to exercise *and* masturbate at the same time—in public— without anyone being the wiser? All you need are a couple of well-placed accessories! Wear Luna Beads (see page 109) or a We-Vibe (see page 104) under your clothes. Luna Beads offer subtle pleasure when you move, dance, exercise, or jog, and each little hit of pleasure reminds you to do your pelvic floor exercises. The We-Vibe is a vibrator that rests against your clitoris and G-spot. It's remote-controlled, so that you can monitor the intensity and type of sensations (such as constant pulsing or roller-coaster pulse patterns). Just hide the remote in your pocket after you switch it up: No one will suspect that pleasure is on your mind.

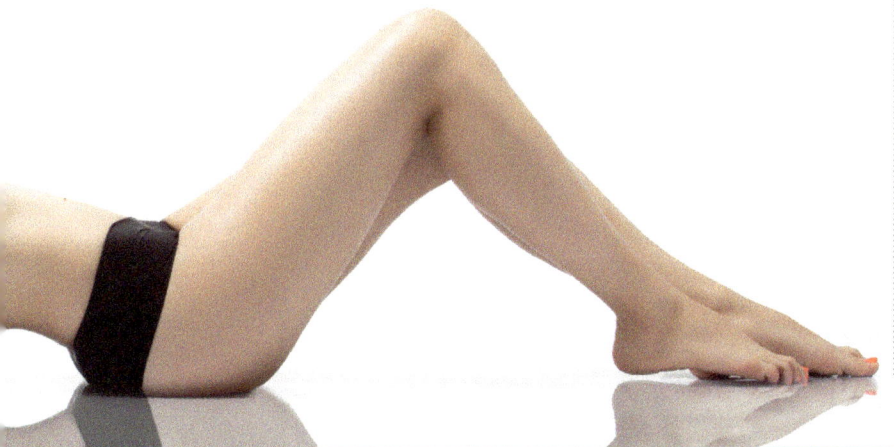

» RELAX YOUR LEGS. Most of us are inclined to squeeze our legs together when we're close to orgasm because it just feels so good. But doing this can actually diminish the power of your orgasm. That's because there's nowhere for your muscles to contract further with the orgasm when they're already contracted! Go ahead and squeeze your legs—just be sure to relax them afterward, as you would with pelvic floor or Kegel exercises. If you're a regular squeezer, you can change the habit by relaxing on every outbreath. That way, if you tense up again, another tension-releasing outbreath is just around the corner. Remaining tense for more than a few breaths means you'll experience only a slight increase in pleasure, which will dissipate quickly. Relaxing in between squeezes lets you amass even more erotic energy before the big O happens, which means the big O will be even stronger. Like any new habit, it might feel a little weird at first, but the payoff—bigger and better orgasms—is so worth it.

» STIMULATE LOTS OF PLEASURE POINTS. Oh, the joys of being pleasured by multiple hands at once! But that's tough to achieve when the only hands nearby are your own. That's where toys come in: They can often work hands-free, providing you with extra stimulation when you're on your own. Vibrating or non-vibrating nipple clamps, for example, can yield either gentle or intense nipple sensations, leaving your hands free to do other exciting things. Or try a butt plug: It's designed to stay in place (with or without vibration) so that you can enjoy the pleasure effortlessly. Lying on your stomach, you can grind your clit against a vibrator or pillow while your hands roam elsewhere. You can also strap a dildo to a chair or suction it to a wall, and thrust onto it while you use your hands to play with your clitoris. Whichever way you do it, the more erogenous zones you engage at once, the more explosive the sensations and finale will be.

» BE A TEASE. Teasing—that is, building your arousal levels, then backing off—is a great way to lengthen your solo sex session. Sure, teasing yourself is a little harder than being teased by a partner, because once you get close to the final destination, so to speak, you just want to *get* there already! But if you can manage it, it works wonders. Especially if you haven't been able to have multiple orgasms (yet! See chapter 7 to find out how), teasing can make your solo play last longer. After all, you went to all the trouble of snagging some private time for yourself, then getting relaxed and into the mood, so maybe a longer pleasure session will feel more worthwhile than a shorter one. Teasing yourself by backing off when your arousal is high and transferring your

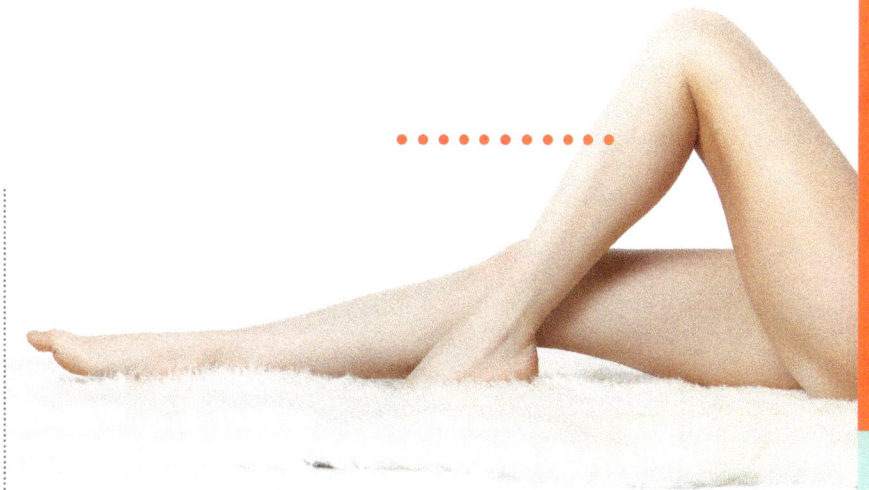

focus to another erogenous zone means you'll enjoy more pleasure throughout the encounter, plus a bigger blast at the end. For example, if you're playing with your clitoris and you feel your arousal nearing its peak, move away from your clit and give your labia a little love instead. Don't wait until the last minute to back off, though: You might tip yourself over the edge into orgasm and lose the momentum you gained. (The closer to orgasm you get, the harder it is to stop.) Back off when you know you'll be able to switch gears without losing your focus entirely. And then build again by stimulating a different erogenous zone.

» TAKE YOUR TIME. If you can orgasm within just a few minutes using fingers or toys, or both, that's fantastic. But if you give yourself a little more time, your body will be able to accumulate more erotic energy before you come. You'll probably come harder, and you'll enjoy the buildup of pleasure as well! So, try using your vibrator at a lower speed, or spend a little more time around your labia rather than going straight for the clit. Use your favorite slow-but-sure technique instead of that race-to-the-finish trick that works so well. If you can stretch out your arousal from three to six minutes, or from ten to twenty minutes or more, you'll find that the end result is much more powerful. Don't look at the clock, though! Tease yourself, and explore your body's different erogenous zones: that'll help you take your time.

Don't feel you have to try all these suggestions at once—if you do that, you'll just end up thinking too much instead of focusing on the pleasure. Experiment with them one at a time, and soon you'll have a whole arsenal of pleasure options at your disposal. And that means better orgasms, too! Chapter 7 will show you exactly how to get there.

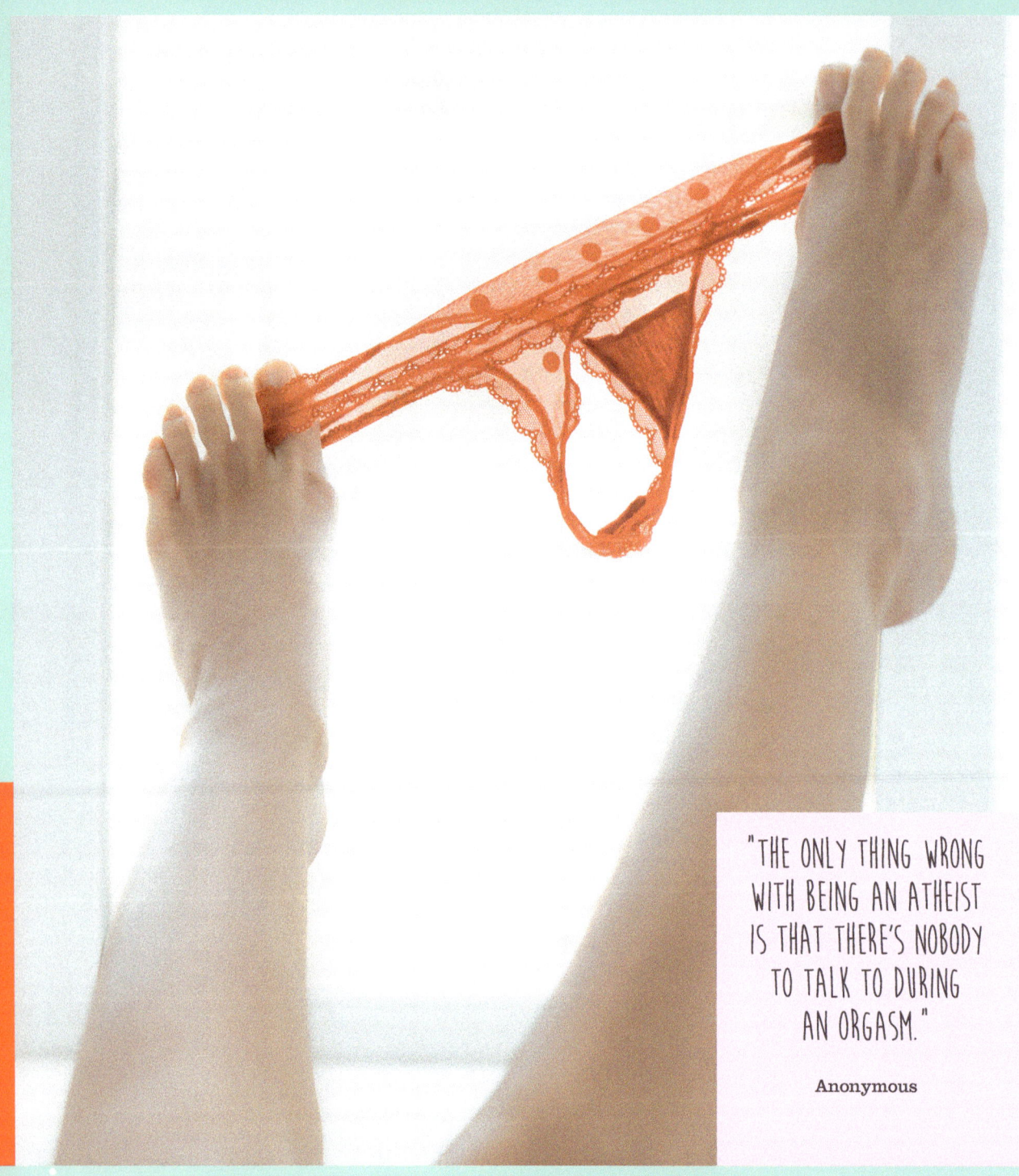

"THE ONLY THING WRONG WITH BEING AN ATHEIST IS THAT THERE'S NOBODY TO TALK TO DURING AN ORGASM."

Anonymous

BIGGER, BETTER,
MULTIPLE
ORGASMS

7

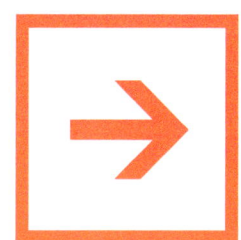

La petite mort. The Big O. Climax. Whichever way you like to say it, an orgasm is a special experience that usually happens at the middle or end of the (solo or partnered) erotic adventure. But are they really the earth-shaking experiences depicted in Hollywood films or in mainstream porn? What do orgasms look like, and how do they happen? Some of us discover them by accident, while others work hard at achieving them. Some women might not have experienced them at all, or aren't sure whether they have or not. And that's perfectly fine. Orgasm isn't the only way to conclude a great solo sex session, and it's not the only reason to enjoy solo play. Sure, it's true that orgasms feel great: they offer a lovely buildup of pressure and pleasure followed by the satisfaction of release and relaxation. But erotic pleasure is individual and every woman will arrive at orgasm in her own way and in her own time, so it's important not to focus too much on the grand finale. After all, pleasure feels good, whether you have an orgasm during it or not! In this chapter, you'll learn everything you need to know about orgasms—how they happen, why they happen—and what you can do to make them happen as often as possible.

PLEASURE AS A JOURNEY

When it comes to sex, it's easy to overemphasize orgasm. We tend to think of it as the Holy Grail of pleasure, but that can be self-defeating. See, when you're having sex, solo or partnered, your body is in "rest and digest" mode: you're relaxed, your blood is circulating freely (especially to your erogenous zones!), and you're present in the moment. But becoming even a little bit anxious about whether orgasm will happen or not can switch your body into "fight or flight" mode. Suddenly, blood circulates away from your erogenous zones to your muscles and vital organs, shallow breathing ensues, and your focus shifts to fear of the future rather than the sensations you're enjoying right now. And that means orgasm becomes even less possible or probable. What all this

means is, the key to having an orgasm is not thinking about the orgasm. Instead, stay present in the process by simply experiencing and enjoying erotic pleasure, and don't focus on orgasm as a goal. (Of course, that's a little like telling a friend "Don't think about bears" when you're hiking in the woods, and then actually expecting her *not* to think about bears! Still, though, imagining pleasure as a journey and focusing on the wonderful sensations you're experiencing right now is the first step you need to take to maximize your erotic potential, whether you have an orgasm or not.)

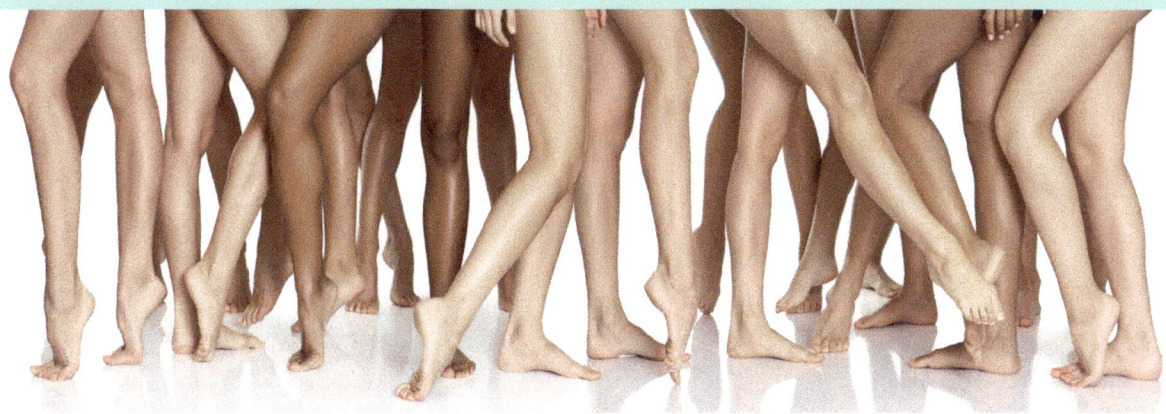

ORGASM Q&A

WHAT IS AN ORGASM, ANYWAY?

It's tough to describe, but an orgasm is a physical experience that's often compared to a really, really good sneeze: it involves a buildup of tension that culminates in a spasmodic release of pressure, and the result is a sensation of relief and relaxation that occurs as the body releases oxytocin and prolactin. During an incomplete orgasm—which is like a sneeze that didn't quite happen—the tension gradually subsides, but this happens too slowly to result in any sense of satisfaction or pleasure.

Here's what's going on physiologically: During arousal, blood fills your erectile tissue, and your heart rate rises, in the same way that it does when you exercise. Arousal builds, and your body is flooded with endorphins (which give you the ability to handle much more pain than usual, as well as pleasure). Then orgasm happens. It's a series of contractions of the pelvic floor muscles, and these contractions usually occur about 0.8 seconds apart. This sequence of contractions lasts five to twenty seconds, or even longer. Some people can feel each individual contraction, while others just experience an overall sense of pleasure. Afterward, your blood drains from the erectile tissue, your clitoris might become extra-sensitive, and your breathing and heart rate will slow down—unless, of course, you build up arousal again!

SHE'S GOING THE DISTANCE.

The longest recorded female orgasm was forty-three seconds long, and included twenty-five contractions. There have likely been many non-recorded orgasms that go even farther longer, but who has time to count?

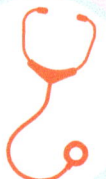

TOO MUCH OF A GOOD THING

If you suffer from Persistent Genital Arousal Disorder (PGAD), you'll experience uncontrollable arousal that's unrelated to sexual desire. Arousal can occur at any time, can last for days or even weeks, and may or may not lead to orgasm. Having an orgasm every five minutes—literally!—might sound great, but most people who have PGAD would prefer not to, because it can be very distracting and even painful.

TYPES OF ORGASM

The truth is, there are as many types of orgasms as there are people in the world: each person's experience is different. But, according to a study published in 2011 in the *Journal of Sexual Medicine*, there are four major nerves that travel from the genitals to the brain. They are:

» Pudendal nerve, which connects to the clitoris

» Pelvic nerve, which connects to the vagina

» Hypogastric nerve, which connects to the cervix and uterus

» Vagus nerve, which connects to the cervix and uterus, bypassing the spinal cord

Women have experienced orgasm as a result of all kinds of pleasure: vaginal stimulation, including G-spot, cervical, A-spot, and perineal stimulation, as well as anal stimulation, squeezing the pelvic muscles, nipples, kissing, or even "thinking off" (that is, without touching themselves at all). Some women orgasm in their sleep, even if they can't come while they're awake. Other women who have little or no sensation in the pelvic area due to paralysis have experienced orgasm via the vagus nerve. The point is, there are plenty of ways to come, and everyone responds differently; remember that it's not a competition to see who can orgasm in the most creative way! Practice your solo sex skills to figure out what gives you pleasure, *then* explore new techniques for getting to the big finish.

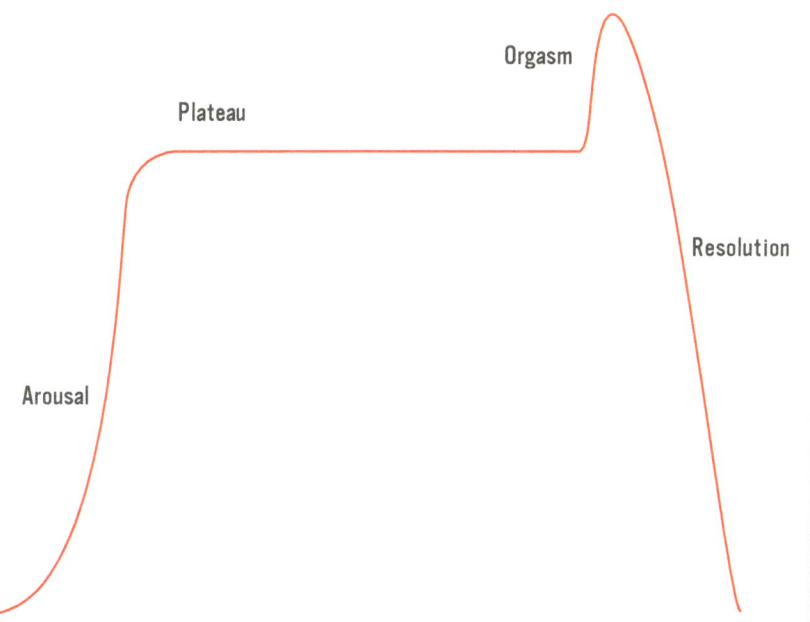

Orgasm

Plateau

Resolution

Arousal

THE POWER OF THE VAGUS NERVE

In one study, five women with spinal cord injuries who were paralyzed from the lower torso down used toys to stimulate their vaginas. These women had been told that they would never experience genital sensation again. In this study, however, the women felt pleasure as well as pain blockage. Three of them experienced orgasm. The study concluded that the vagus nerve, which bypasses the spinal cord, conducted the pleasurable signals to the brain.

THE PHASES OF ORGASM

This is an image of a common arousal pattern, originally created by sexologists William H. Masters and Virginia E. Johnson in 1966. These days, it's often criticized for being outdated and because it doesn't take into account the vast number of factors that can affect arousal. But it's still very helpful when it comes to understanding the process of orgasm.

First up is the arousal stage. Erotic touch and sexy thoughts cause your genital area to fill with blood, your heart rate steadily increases, and desire for more pleasure builds. Eventually, you reach a point where your physical arousal doesn't increase, but remains relatively constant as you continue to feel pleasure; this is the second stage. It's really important to stay focused when you reach this plateau—but, unfortunately, this is where a lot of us get stuck. Now is when you might start to criticize the way in which your body is responding, and you might begin to get anxious: Why isn't it happening *now*? Will it happen at all? Why can't I come in the same way all the women's magazines describe it? How can all my friends or partner's exes come at the drop of a hat, and here I am taking *forever*?

Or distractions might creep in: How much time do I have before I pick up the kids? Can I get around to repainting the bathroom next week? Suddenly, it's hard to focus, and you don't feel very aroused anymore. Eventually, you're likely to give up, get bored, or decide to try again another time as the arousal plummets. But when you focus on the pleasure instead of distractions or critical thoughts, you'll stay in that pleasure plateau, and you're more likely to reach the next stage of arousal: orgasm.

Orgasm lasts between three and twenty seconds, or sometimes more, and consists of rhythmic contractions followed by the resolution phase, during which arousal decreases very quickly, and you feel relaxed and sated.

HOW DO I KNOW WHETHER I HAD AN ORGASM?

The standard answer to this question is, "You'd know if you did!" But that is actually not necessarily true. Lots of people wonder whether they've already had orgasms or may even be having them without even knowing it, because orgasms can be elusive little devils. And if you watch women having orgasms in porn films (or in the famous scene from *When Harry Met Sally* in which Sally, played by Meg Ryan, loudly fakes an orgasm in a restaurant), then you might have gotten the idea that all orgasms produce shrieks and full-body convulsions. The truth is that orgasms can often be much more subtle in expression. So, how do you know? One clue is clitoral oversensitivity: After orgasm, the clitoris becomes suddenly

and intensely sensitive to touch, so much so that you'd push a partner's hand, mouth, or penis away from it. Other types of orgasm don't usually result in the same kind of sensitivity, although most leave you with a sudden and pleasurable feeling of release (like the relief you feel after a sneeze), followed by deep relaxation. Some orgasms make you want to fall asleep afterward, while others make you want to keep on going! The way in which you respond to an orgasm is completely unique, and depends on factors like your energy levels and the type of orgasm you just had. To sum up, you might not know whether you're having an orgasm when you're in the moment, but if your clitoris is super-sensitive afterward and you feel relaxed and sated, then the answer is probably yes.

WHAT IF I DON'T ORGASM?

First of all, know that you've got plenty of company. A *lot* of women don't orgasm, and some don't learn how until they're in their forties, fifties, or beyond. And that can be incredibly frustrating: it can add stress to your relationship with your partner (not to mention your relationship with yourself), and it can make self-pleasure a less-than-exciting task. It can make you feel as if you're "broken," so to speak, and it might even be the reason you're reading this book. (If you're looking for more resources, *The Elusive Orgasm* by Vivienne Cass is a great book, and can also help you work toward orgasm.) But whether you're having orgasms or not, please remember that sex, solo or otherwise, can still offer a lot of pleasure and joy. Lots of women find they enjoy sex much more when they think of pleasure as a journey instead of a destination. And sometimes simply freeing ourselves of the pressure and emphasis we place on orgasm can help us get there.

If you don't orgasm, asking yourself a few important questions might help you understand what's getting in your way:

1. How do you feel about masturbation in general? Does the idea turn you on or off? Make you excited or feel disgusted? Do you think it's a good use of time, or is it time wasted? Negative associations with solo play can stop you from experiencing pleasure during it.

2. Have you used the diagram in chapter 2 to help you explore your vulva, vagina, and other erogenous zones? Have you tried lots of the techniques in chapter 4? What did you learn or notice? Even if some of the techniques didn't float your boat at the time, experimenting with different types of strokes does expand your pleasure options. Sometimes what didn't work yesterday will feel great today—perhaps with a little variation in depth, pressure, or location. Go ahead and explore your own body, if you haven't already: understanding what's going on "down there" can help you embrace pleasure more fully. And you need to do it more than once—maybe even ten or twenty times!

3. Have you tried using physical or psychological tools to help you get there? Lube? A vibrator (such as the Original Magic Wand)? Fantasizing about a sex scenario you'd love to try? Many women find that lube, toys, or fantasy—or even all three at once!—are integral to solo sex satisfaction. Even if you don't end up using them forever, these tools can help you orgasm the first few times, until your body learns how to let go and surrender to the orgasm.

4. When you have solo sex, do you hear a "negative monologue" in your head—one that judges you or your performance, or suggests you're doing something immoral or wrong? If so, know that you can overpower those negative messages with positive ones, like the mantra in chapter 3. Repeating positive messages to yourself reinforces them, and once you believe them, you'll be better able to notice and enjoy the pleasure solo play offers.

5. Do you give up after five minutes? Ten? Twenty? Don't! It can take more than thirty minutes for you to reach orgasm. If you get bored, or feel frustrated that you're not making enough "progress," try to let go of the goal. Use a toy to help you build arousal. Set a timer for 30 minutes (or more), and make a deal with yourself: During that time, you're only allowed to do pleasurable things. Even if you end up simply touching or stroking parts of your body, devote that time to your own pleasure.

6. Do you focus on what's going wrong, or on what you "should" be feeling or doing, rather than on what feels good? If so, you might get frustrated more easily, and that'll only make you feel more anxious. Instead of paying attention to what isn't working, focus on what *is*. Notice and congratulate yourself when you feel pleasure: that's progress! Celebrate the small victories (which are actually big ones in disguise): staying present, feeling new sensations, trying something new. And don't expect a specific type of response from your body! Everyone responds to pleasure in different ways.

7. Do you get distracted by everyday thoughts, like home renovations, what to cook for dinner, or other things that aren't related to arousal? That's okay. Gently bring yourself back to the present moment, and to the lovely sensations your body is experiencing. Remind yourself to focus on the pleasure.

Whether you orgasm or not, it's important to be aware of your thoughts, body sensations, and emotions during solo sex. Which of the above questions resonate with you? During your next masturbation session, notice what's going on in both your body and your mind. Then reflect on it in your journal, with a friend, or with a therapist. Awareness is the first step toward change!

WHAT STOPS ME FROM REACHING ORGASM?

Whether you get there in lots of different ways, one way, or not at all, a number of things can make climaxing more difficult, including the following.

» MEDICATIONS. The birth control pill can make you less likely to orgasm, and the same goes for antidepressants (SSRIs), which can wreak havoc on your ability to orgasm even after you've stopped taking the meds. (Personal anecdotes suggest that Wellbutrin seems to have fewer negative effects on orgasm than other drugs in this category.) If you take any kind of medication regularly, check its side effects, and talk to your doctor: some folks are more sensitive to medications and their side effects than others. You might be able to try an alternative medication with fewer undesired consequences.

» HORMONES. Becoming aroused and reaching orgasm can be easier at certain times of the menstrual cycle. Usually, it's easiest when you're ovulating, but some women have more success right before or during their period. Pregnancy can also make you more or less likely to orgasm, depending upon the individual; you might try a different type of stimulation than whatever works for you when you're not pregnant, or if you're breast-feeding, add some extra lube (because breast-feeding tends to dry up the natural moisture in your vagina). What all this means is, in general, hormonal fluctuations may make it harder to come.

» DISTRACTIONS. When you're having solo sex, do you worry that someone might walk in and interrupt you? Do you worry about what your mother, kids, or partner would think if they knew what you were doing right now? Are you making a list of all the chores you *still* haven't gotten around to? When your mind wanders like this, you remove yourself from the pleasure of the present moment. The result: arousal wanes and drifts away.

» BODY IMAGE AND SELF-ESTEEM. Your attitude toward yourself can have a huge impact on whether or not you can reach orgasm. Are you feeling great about your work life, your relationships with your partner, friends, and family, your body and fitness level, and your life in general? If the answer is yes, then you're more likely to be able to come. But if you feel unmotivated at work or school, frustrated with your partner, or disappointed with your level of fitness, or are dealing with a recent trauma, your orgasms may not be as frequent or as strong as they could be.

» STRESS. If you're stressed about your job, relationships, finances, family, illness, kids, or just about anything else, then it's likely that your orgasmic potential will suffer as a result. But solo sex can be a great (safe, healthy) way to escape those worries for a few minutes. Some people are able to step away from those stressors and soak up some much-need pleasure through solo play. (If you're already one of those people, I salute you!)

» PRESSURE TO PERFORM. You already know that placing pressure on yourself to orgasm can backfire in a big way. Well, you're also less likely to come if you're pressuring yourself to orgasm in a certain way, from a particular type of stimulation, or within a specified time frame.

» RESENTMENT. If you resent the fact that your partner or friends or porn performers have a way easier time than you do when it comes to pleasure, then your emotional state will negatively impact your focus and ability to do the very thing that you are trying to achieve.

» TIREDNESS. When you're focusing all your energy on staying awake, it's possible that solo pleasure is the last thing you want to think about. Plus, tired sex is usually lazy sex, which means that your orgasm will probably be less than ecstatic. But if you can orgasm easily with fingers, and use a toy or technique that makes orgasm effortless, you'll probably have a better experience—even if you're exhausted.

» ATTITUDES, IDEAS, AND BELIEFS ABOUT SOLO SEX. If you're convinced that touching yourself is gross, dirty, or sinful, then you'll find it really hard to get aroused, which means you probably won't orgasm (or if you do, it won't be terribly exciting). And sometimes we internalize those negative ideas so deeply that we don't even realize they're there. Intellectually, you might believe that solo sex is a perfectly respectable, valuable activity, but your body might be responding to hidden feelings of shame. Pay attention to your "gut" feelings. Do you feel tense or reluctant when it comes to solo sex?

» LOW TESTOSTERONE LEVELS. Yes, women's bodies produce testosterone, too, and low levels of testosterone can mean a lower sex drive and more difficulty reaching orgasm. Your doctor can test your testosterone levels, and, if necessary, advise you on natural and prescription remedies.

» DRUGS AND ALCOHOL. Plenty of people feel that a glass or two of wine or a little bit of marijuana can help them relax. That's partly true. These substances lower your inhibitions, so that you don't care so much about the little voice in your head that's judging or criticizing you as you touch yourself. Don't misunderstand this as an endorsement of drug use or regular drinking, though. In fact, if you've noticed that you're more able to enjoy pleasure when you're under the influence, then take some time to examine your beliefs about your body, sex, and masturbation—and find other ways to relax and let go rather than relying on those substances. Besides, consuming more than one or two units of alcohol before solo or partnered sex is completely counterproductive, because it dulls your senses and makes it harder for you to be receptive to any kind of pleasure.

» POOR CIRCULATION. If your circulation isn't great, then your body might have a tough time pumping blood to your erogenous zones—and that's essential to arousal and pleasure. Try having solo sex after a workout, when your heart rate has already been increased, and when your blood is really zooming through your veins. Plus, exercise can help you relax and focus, and it boosts energy and self-esteem.

» NOTHING FEELS THAT GOOD. Of course, if you're having a hard time getting aroused, orgasm will be improbable, if not impossible. Try upping your arousal by using toys, practicing your breathing, indulging in a delicious fantasy—anything that turns you on. Check out the suggestions in chapter 4 for more inspiration.

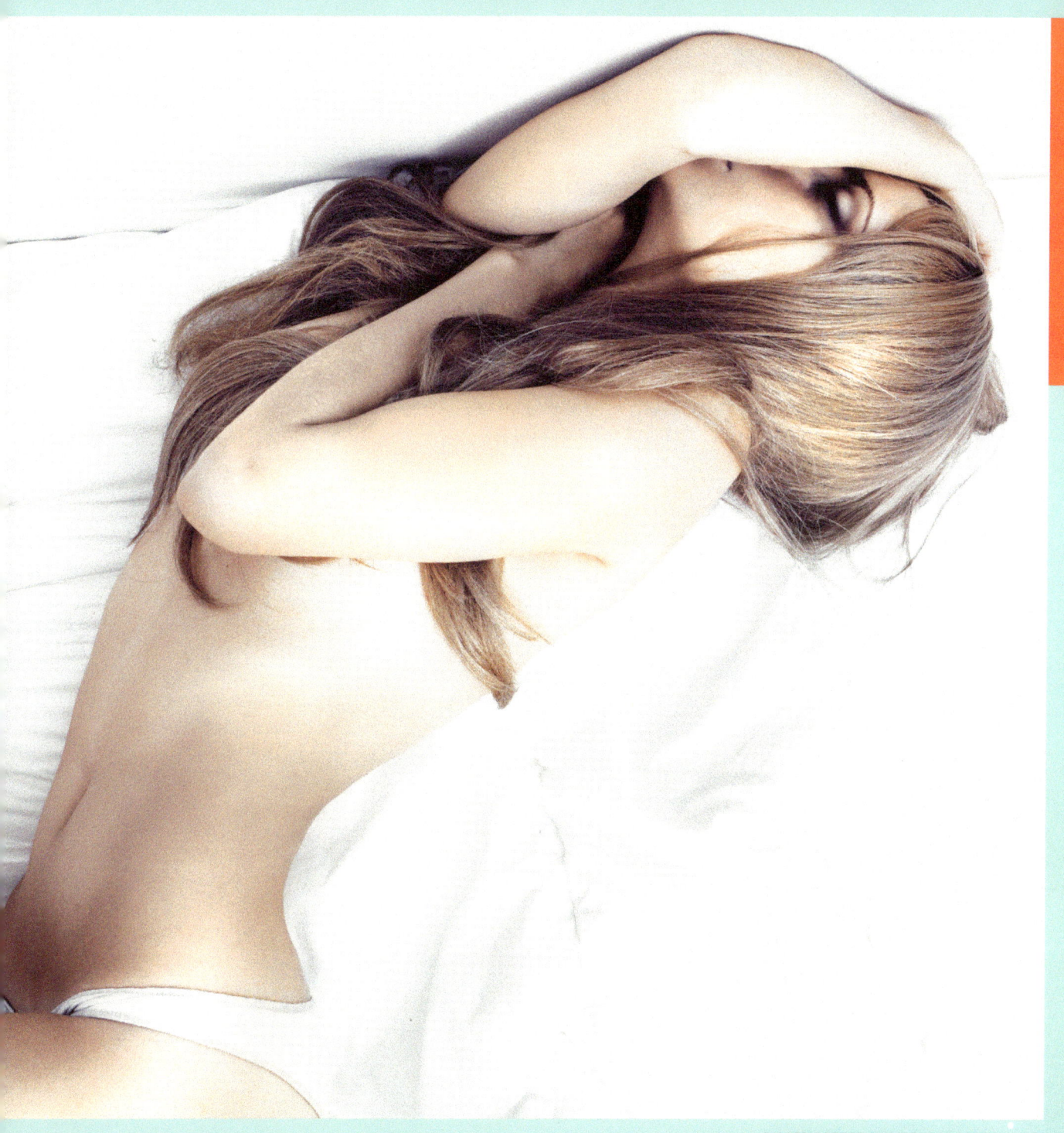

WHAT IF I'M STUCK ON THE EDGE AND CAN'T COME?

Lots of women feel like they're "almost there," but can't quite nudge themselves over the edge into orgasm. Here are a few ways to help yourself get there. Focus on the ones that speak to you.

» Savor the moment like a chocolate truffle: See how intensely you can experience pleasure.

» Write it down. Keep a log of your thoughts and emotions as you pleasure yourself. Over time, tune in to any patterns that might emerge.

» Focus on the sensations that you actually feel, rather than on what you think you "should" be feeling.

» Notice which sensations you're pushing away and why. Consider exploring this with a trusted friend or a sex-positive therapist.

» Surrender your mind to your body: Go where your body wants to take you, rather than where you think it is supposed to go, and allow yourself to receive pleasure.

» Increase the intensity of stimulation. Try using a powerful vibrator, especially if you're getting bored and your fingers or your usual vibrator can't offer more power.

» Breathe, and let yourself make sounds. Don't be shy: Sometimes you can even fake it 'til you make it!

» Rhythm is king. Our bodies respond to a rhythm of pleasure: up and down, side to side, or around and around. Stick with it, and don't switch it up too much.

» Move. Don't stay in the same spot, especially when you're using a powerful vibrator. Our bodies perceive difference, so if you don't move your fingers or your vibrator a little, you'll become numb to the pleasure.

» Let go of the focus on orgasm. Give yourself permission to feel pleasure, and let the orgasm present itself in its own time.

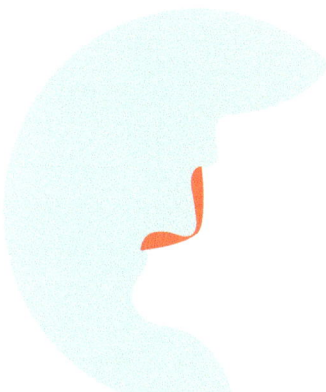

IMPROVING YOUR ORGASMS

There are both psychological and physical strategies that can help you make your orgasms longer, more intense, and more satisfying.

RELAX

Psychologically, the most important thing you can do to have better, more frequent orgasms is simply to relax. As I mentioned earlier in this chapter, you need to be in "rest and digest" mode—not "fight or flight" mode—to enjoy ultimate pleasure. Of course, that's easier said than done! There's no magic pill that ensures complete relaxation (if only!), but there are things you can do to chill out.

Let's start with breathing. Taking deep breaths triggers the vagus nerve, part of the parasympathetic "rest and digest" nervous system that controls your relaxation response. So, put your hands on your tummy, and focus on the way in which your hands move up and down with each breath. Breathe in through the nose and out through the mouth to form a "circle" of respiration. If it helps, you might want to visualize stress leaving your body. What does it look like to you?

Similarly, positive thinking can calm you down and decrease stress levels. Recite a mantra or listen to a CD with a positive message. Or visualize a beach, a cool, shady forest, or another peaceful scene. Some people find prayer to be calming and uplifting, while others choose meditation. Because meditation features in so many different traditions, from Buddhism to nonreligious forms of yoga, you'll be able to practice a version that's in keeping with your beliefs. Alternatively, engage your mind by reading something inspiring that speaks to you, such as the Tao Te Ching, the writing of Mahatma Gandhi, the poetry of Rumi, speeches by Martin Luther King, or any uplifting or spiritual text that you connect with.

You might also consider self-hypnosis. Visit a hypnosis practitioner, who'll be able to teach you simple self-hypnosis techniques that'll help you calm your mind, especially before sex. And approaching sex with a calm, open mind is ideal, because that means you'll be able to stay in the present, focusing on all five of your senses from arousal right through orgasm.

And you don't need to sit still to be chill. Movement can help you tune in to where you are in the here and now. So make time for that workout, kick a ball around with the kids, go for a walk, or attend a yoga class. If you're short on time, get off the bus a few stops earlier: Walking a bit can help you feel more centered. Or shut the bedroom door, turn up the tunes, and dance (yes, alone!). Let your body follow the music, and don't judge the quality or style of your dancing. Pre- or post-dance, mindful stretching can help, too; be sure to focus on your muscles and your breathing instead of letting your mind wander to to-do lists. And remember the progressive relaxation exercise from chapter 3? It's a fabulous way to relax your entire body from head to toe—

literally. Start with your toes: squeeze them tight for five seconds, then relax them for five seconds. Repeat the process with your feet, calves, thighs, and so on, until you reach your face. It takes just two minutes, and your body will feel way more relaxed than it did before you began.

Making time to express yourself is another way to unwind. If you enjoy writing, then do some journaling: Putting preoccupying thoughts on paper helps you work through them, so the writing process can be cathartic and relaxing as well as a form of creative expression. Or, if you're not into writing, just write down a list of all the things you need to do, with timelines for each. Once you have a plan, you'll be able to relax, knowing that you've already thought about how to get it all done. You could also take an hour to cross something off that to-do list: de-cluttering, for example. (Just be sure to stick to a manageable goal: don't try to reorganize the entire basement or paint the whole house!)

And, as always, allow yourself time to do something you love, whether it's drawing, writing, researching, reading, baking, collecting stamps—you name it.

STAY SELF-AWARE

If staying relaxed is vital to great solo sex and satisfying orgasms, so is being aware of your thoughts and emotions, especially the way you feel about your own body. That's because awareness helps us better understand our experiences, and improve on them. In the same way that you might have developed certain habits unconsciously, you may also have developed patterns of arousal that work against or inhibit you from fully embracing pleasure. These patterns may be so familiar that you might not know they exist until you stop and notice them. That's why it's important to be aware of how we become aroused. So, during solo sex, pay attention to:

» THOUGHTS THAT GO THROUGH YOUR MIND ABOUT SEX, PLEASURE, AND YOUR BODY. Is that little voice in your head repeating negative ideas about your appearance, your body's responses, or the kinds of pleasure or fantasies that you enjoy? When it comes to orgasm, are you placing heavy expectations on yourself about the way in which you "should" come? Keep a notebook close by so that you can write things down (it's not as distracting as it sounds: after jotting your thoughts down, you can forget about them and move back to the pleasure at hand). Later, you can revisit your thoughts and try to let go of them through journaling or talking to a sex-positive friend or therapist.

» YOUR MIND WANDERING. Notice whether your mind tends to drift toward non-erotic things, such as work responsibilities or grocery shopping. This often leads to your pleasure levels dropping during the plateau phase. Don't get down on yourself, just gently bring yourself back to the moment.

» DISTRACTIONS. Getting distracted by noises from next door or worried about who might walk in? Next time, find a quieter, more private place or time for your erotic adventure.

» PLEASURE. Notice what *actually* feels great, not what you think *should* do the trick. Explore your whole body and pay attention to your responses at different levels of arousal: What feels kind of nice now can deliver ecstasy later if you're able to focus. And, of course, once you know what you like, you'll be able to do it again the next time, whether you're alone or with a partner.

» IMPATIENCE OR BOREDOM. Notice whether you get impatient or bored, especially early on in your arousal. If you're watching the clock or giving up after a few minutes, it's probably because you need more stimulation. Engage all of your senses, and ramp up the intensity levels: use toys as well as fingers, and pay attention to music, lighting, scents, and tastes. When you engage different aspects of your brain, you'll have a fuller experience, and you're more likely to want to remain engaged with it.

» OVERSTIMULATION. If you begin to feel overwhelmed by the sensations, it's probably because you've been distracted, your arousal has begun to flag, and your body can't tolerate or enjoy the same intense pleasure that it could when you were more aroused. Thus, you feel oversensitive, in the same way you would if someone were to touch your clitoris before you were aroused. Reduce the stimulation, and build your arousal back up again.

This might sound like a lot to think about while you're supposed to be enjoying yourself, but don't worry, it's not as difficult as it seems! And it's worth it, because being aware of the issues that arise for you during solo sex can help you break free of thought patterns that might be preventing you from reaching orgasm.

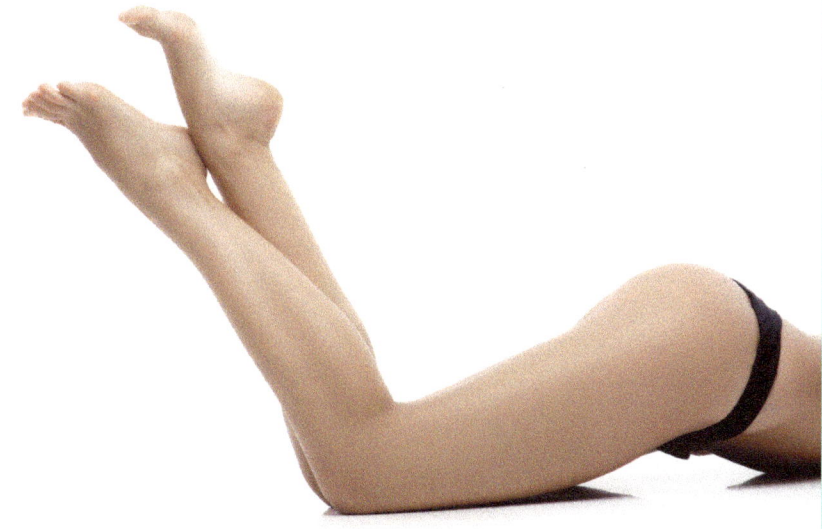

GIVE YOURSELF PERMISSION

Women are exposed to a number of negative stereotypes about what enjoying sexual pleasure means—and, far too often, women who actively pursue sexual pleasure are labeled "sluts," or are considered "selfish" for taking ownership of their sexuality. Aren't "good girls" supposed to wait for a man to take care of them, and to "give" them sexual satisfaction? Even if the rational part of your brain knows this isn't true, sometimes a small part of you still needs to be given permission before you're ready to take charge of your own sexual pleasure.

So, if you feel guilty when it comes to enjoying solo sex, remind yourself that self-pleasure is healthy on a physical level, and it's also vital to stress release and self-care in general. Try using a mantra to help reinforce these positive messages about self-pleasure; chapter 3 can show you how (see page 56). And if you worry that there are more important things to be done, tell yourself that this is time well spent: It's time you set aside for yourself. Because reaching orgasm can take more than a few minutes, allow yourself to be fully present for the entire duration of your solo sex session. Besides, the more pressure you put on yourself to "hurry up," the less likely you are to enjoy yourself.

It's completely okay to use toys during solo sex, too. After all, why shouldn't you do everything you can to make self-pleasure even more satisfying? Some women worry that using toys is improper or "wrong," but there's no such thing as wrong: If it works for you, it's right. Plus, over half of American women use vibrators. If they're all having a good time, why should you miss out? Multiple types of stimulation combined with a little variety can do wonders for your solo sex adventures! The same goes for lubricant. Especially if you're using a toy, adding a little lube just makes everything more comfortable and pleasurable. There's no one around to judge you, so don't worry about what anyone thinks!

And when it comes to the crucial moment—the big O—sometimes we tend to hold ourselves back. Even if you haven't had an orgasm yet and are eager to experience it, you might find yourself pushing it away when you're almost there. I know that doesn't make logical sense, but it's a very real phenomenon that you might not notice until you start paying attention. This reluctance can stem from fear of the unknown, from the desire to wait until you're in the presence of a partner for your "first" or special orgasm, or, simply, from an inability to let go. Those of us with type-A personalities (and you know who you are!) are used to knowing what we want and going for it, which means that letting go and relinquishing control can be tough sometimes. Think about the French phrase for orgasm: *la petite mort*. Translated as "the little death," it symbolizes a letting-go of ego, a sort of temporary death-to-self that happens when you allow the body to take over without giving it conscious direction. To allow the body to do what it instinctively and reflexively knows how to do, you need to get your head out of the way first.

When you do actually orgasm, you might worry that you'll make a mess. Lots of women hold back because they're afraid they might urinate if they come. Although that's technically possible, it is highly improbable, and besides, this type of sensation is usually caused by G-spot stimulation only, and you're unlikely to experience it if you're enjoying other types of stimulation. Breathing deeply through those uncomfortable moments actually helps calm the alarm bell in your head that yells, "You're going to pee!" Nonetheless, you might feel more comfortable when you use the toilet before you start your masturbation session, and then try having solo sex in the shower, or even while you're sitting on the toilet, where you're more likely to be able to let go. If you're holding back because you're afraid of urinating, you're also limiting your response to pleasure. Just let go and enjoy!

SAVOR THE EXPERIENCE

Far too often, we don't approach our daily activities mindfully. For example, imagine you have a box of chocolate truffles to indulge in. (If you don't like truffles, that's okay, think about another favorite food instead.) You *could* eat even the most divine box of truffles while watching TV, talking on the phone, or doing chores without really focusing on the pleasure they're giving you. But then, when the box is empty, you'll probably feel robbed of the experience of eating them, because you weren't really paying attention when you consumed them. Sometimes we have sex in the same way—without being fully attuned to the experience or the pleasure it can offer.

Now imagine that someone's about to give you the *last* chocolate truffle you'll ever eat. You'll never be able to eat another chocolate truffle as long as you live. Ever. Imagine how you'd savor its flavors and textures: the firm outer shell, the soft chocolate inside, what it tastes like on the top, bottom, and sides of your tongue. The truffle-eating experience would last a whole lot longer this way, and you'd be so present within it that you wouldn't notice if elephants were stampeding right outside your window, or if a brass band suddenly invaded your living room. You'd be devoting your full and complete attention to that truffle. This is the type of focus that can maximize your erotic sensations, too. You need to concentrate on how much your body is feeling: your clitoris, your labia, around and inside your vagina, your nipples—even the sweat beading on your forehead, or your chest heaving in and out with each breath. This level of focus keeps you engaged with the pleasure, and you won't have any mental space to let your mind wander or to worry whether the orgasm will happen or not. (If you do notice your attention drifting, gently bring yourself back to the pleasure at hand—without judging yourself.) Not only will you experience pleasure more fully, but you'll also be much more likely to orgasm, and when you do, it might feel like an unexpected gift, because you haven't been pressuring yourself to come. So remind yourself to savor that truffle!

YOUR MIND IS A POWERFUL SEX ORGAN.

At least one study has shown that women who think erotic thoughts and focus on their body sensations during sex have a higher chance of achieving orgasm than those who don't.

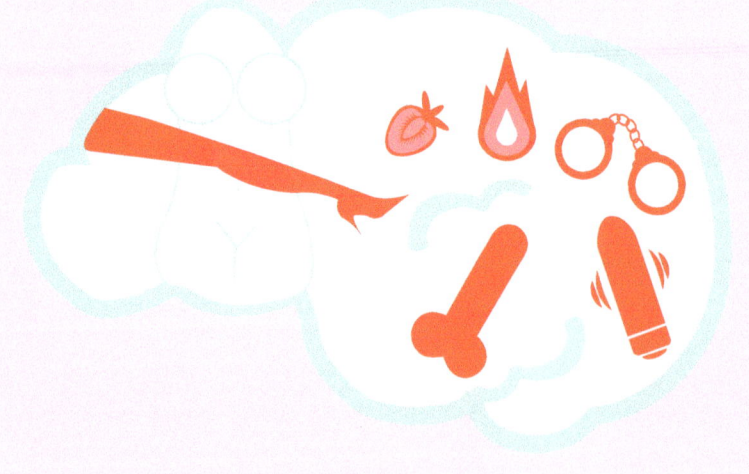

So much of reaching orgasm is psychological, but there are physical strategies that can help you orgasm, too. First, make sure you're comfortable. Door locked? Check. Phone off? Check. Kids, housemates, or parents occupied or out of the house? Check. You'll be much more relaxed—and therefore more aroused—if you're sure that you can play without being disturbed or surprised. Oh, and turn up the heat! It's hard to relax when you're shivering, or when your movement is constrained because you're buried under layers of blankets.

Then, experiment with different erogenous zones. Don some nipple clamps, slide a toy inside your vagina or your butt (or both!), and let both your hands roam wherever they like. The more you have going on, the more all-encompassing the pleasure will be—and the better the orgasm! But don't get too comfortable: Be sure to switch up your pleasure patterns. Just as you need some variety in partner sex play, you need it in solo play, too. Try having solo sex in a different environment (bedroom, bathroom, balcony, office, secluded public area), or at a different time of day (before work, before a date, or after a workout). Try a couple types of stimulation, or indulge in a little fantasy (use some erotica for inspiration, if you like!). Novelty and variety add intensity to the play. Also, you can revisit the strategies for spicing up solo play in chapter 6, including focusing on your breathing, allowing yourself to be vocal, relaxing your legs instead of squeezing them, and drawing out your solo sex romp a little longer. These are all great ways to make climax that much more likely.

And when orgasm does happen, don't stop what you're doing! When you stop pleasuring yourself after orgasm, your arousal plummets, and it'll take a long time to build it up again. Remember the vestibular bulbs—the erectile tissue that's located between the inner and outer labia—that you read about in chapter 2? Well, unlike the clitoris, which becomes oversensitive when stimulated post-orgasm, touching the vestibular bulbs will still feel good even after you've come. Once orgasm sets in, you may want to stop touching yourself completely, but instead, try moving your focus to this pleasurable but less sensitive area. That'll draw out the pleasure—and your orgasm.

HOW TO HAVE MULTIPLE ORGASMS

Are you a one-hit wonder when it comes to clitoral orgasms? If so, you're not alone. Most of us make the mistake of stopping stimulation at the beginning of the orgasm, because the clitoris becomes overly sensitive. But to have another orgasm, you need to continue the stimulation rather than letting it drop completely. (Otherwise, it can be harder to build up to the next one—and it can take a while as well.) So, as soon as the clitoris becomes sensitive during or post-orgasm, continue the pleasure, just move away from the clitoris. Use a little lube to stimulate the vestibular bulbs on the outside of the inner labia, or anywhere else that feels good and not oversensitive. You'll probably notice that your pleasure levels will plateau for around one minute before your arousal skyrockets again. With your arousal higher, you can return more quickly to intense stimulation and the clitoris, and know that the next orgasm is likely around the corner!

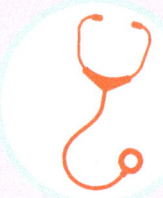

MY DOCTOR SAYS THE G-SPOT DOESN'T EXIST. WHY?

The G-spot remains a hotly debated topic. Many medical professionals still deny its existence, despite the vast number of women whose experiences have demonstrated otherwise. Why? One of the challenges facing the field of sexual research is that much of it is reproduction-focused, and because women can reproduce without experiencing pleasure (not that that's a good thing!), researchers don't pay as much attention to the mechanics of pleasure. Another challenge is the way in which G-spot research is often conducted. It's usually carried out in one of two ways:

» Doctors examine female cadavers in order to find evidence of erectile tissue. This can be problematic, because dead women are often on the older side, and many older folks aren't encouraged to be sexual. That means researchers are less likely to find evidence of healthy tissue in an older woman. (Plus, it's really hard to witness the G-spot in action unless your research subject is actually alive!)

» Studies ask women directly whether they feel pleasure in the G-spot area. That's a good idea, but this method would be much more valid and informative if it were preceded by an educational segment in which women (and their partners) could learn more about where the G-spot is, how to stimulate it, and what might prevent them from finding it in the first place. Think of it this way: You're probably aware that you have a liver, but I bet you've got no idea where it is or what touching it feels like. Similarly, just because you might have heard of the G-spot doesn't mean you automatically know how to find it.

Because medical professionals are trained to listen to traditional research outcomes like these, it makes sense that many doctors would be pretty skeptical of the G-spot's existence, and wouldn't bother even to look for it. But that doesn't mean it doesn't exist: Plenty of women I've met over the years have done their own research, and know better!

WHAT ABOUT G-SPOT ORGASMS?

Once you locate it, the G-spot can be an incredible source of pleasure—if you're into it. Some women love G-spot stimulation, and others think it's overrated. As with all erogenous zones, the way you respond to it is completely individual, so if G-spot pleasure doesn't do anything for you, that's fine! Explore a little first, though, to help you decide.

In order to orgasm from G-spot pleasure, you need to learn about your own G-spot first. Where is it most sensitive? Which style of pressure do you like: a "come hither" motion, a windshield-wiper stroke, a "peace sign" stroke (similar to a "come hither" motion, but with the two fingers spread slightly apart), or firm pressure, as if you were ringing a doorbell? Do you like it shallow or deep? A lot of pressure, or just a little? Do you like to combine it with other types of stimulation? Do you prefer fingers, a soft toy, or a hard toy? Do your preferences change as your arousal increases? Once you understand your preferences, you'll be able to build toward G-spot orgasms.

DOES "SQUIRTING" MEAN I'VE HAD A G-SPOT ORGASM?

This is a common misconception. Not all G-spot orgasms necessarily involve squirting. They're two separate events (for men as well as women, actually!). It's true that most women who ejaculate—and that's about 15 to 20 percent of women—usually do so as a result of G-spot stimulation at the point of orgasm, but it doesn't happen that way for everyone. Some women ejaculate when they have orgasms of any kind. Some women who can't orgasm still ejaculate when aroused. And most women who orgasm, even as a result of G-spot play, don't ejaculate. To make a long story short, the "squirting" response is separate from orgasm, but the two responses sometimes occur simultaneously.

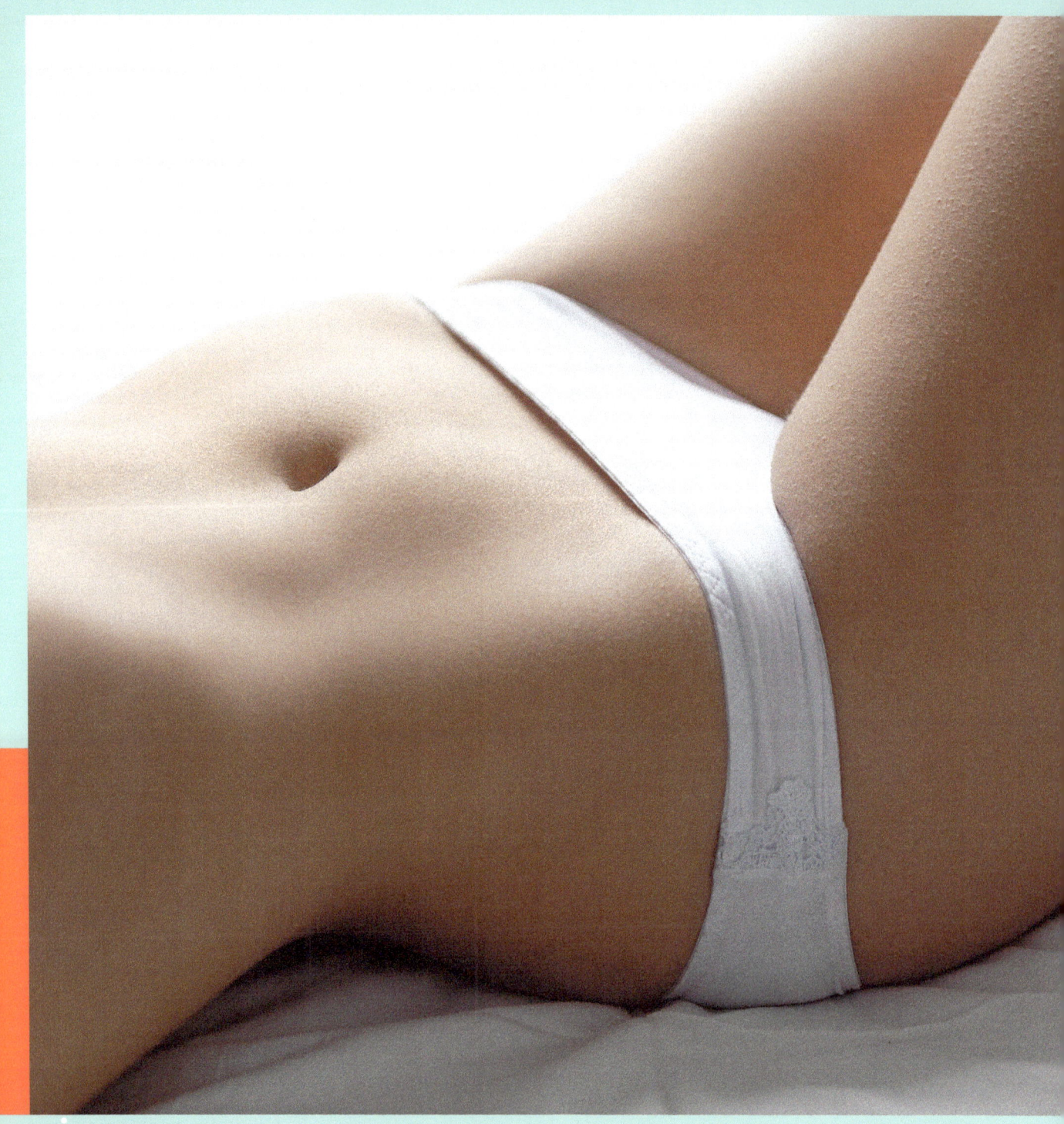

TWO PATHS TO A G-SPOT ORGASM

As a sex educator, I'm often asked, "How do I have a G-spot orgasm?" Before we get into that, let's be very clear on one thing. Forget what you've read by Freud: No single type of orgasm is superior to another. However you get there is the right way. And there's nothing wrong with adding some clit play to penetration or G-spot pleasure. (Most women do! Remember that 70 percent of women need clitoral stimulation in order to orgasm.) And being in the female superior position—that is, "on top"—is the easiest way for most women to orgasm during intercourse. That's because grinding your clitoris against your partner's pubic bone is easily done from this position.

If you do want to learn how to come from G-spot play, these two strategies might help. (Most prefer to start with the first one—you'll soon find out why!) And, if you already orgasm from G-spot stimulation, or if you're not interested in G-spot play but are curious about another way to climax, know that the process is the same, just replace the word "G-spot" with the new type of pleasure you hope to orgasm from.

STRATEGY 1: MULTITASK

» Step 1. Pleasure yourself by playing with your clitoris (or however you usually achieve orgasm). At the same time, pleasure yourself by stimulating your G-spot—or any other erogenous zone you hope will bring you to orgasm. Do this throughout most of the arousal. When your arousal has reached a plateau and you're really close to orgasm, stop the clitoral play and stimulate the G-spot alone. If you orgasm at this point, move on to step 2. If not, try step 1 again until you're able to come after switching to your G-spot. (If you repeat step 1 multiple times with no success, you might try switching to Strategy 2.)

» Step 2. Begin step 1, but this time, stop the clitoral stimulation a little earlier on in your arousal than you did the first time: You're teaching your body to build up arousal from this newer, G-spot-based type of play. If that works, repeat the process, stopping clitoral stimulation and switching to G-spot play a little earlier in your arousal each time.

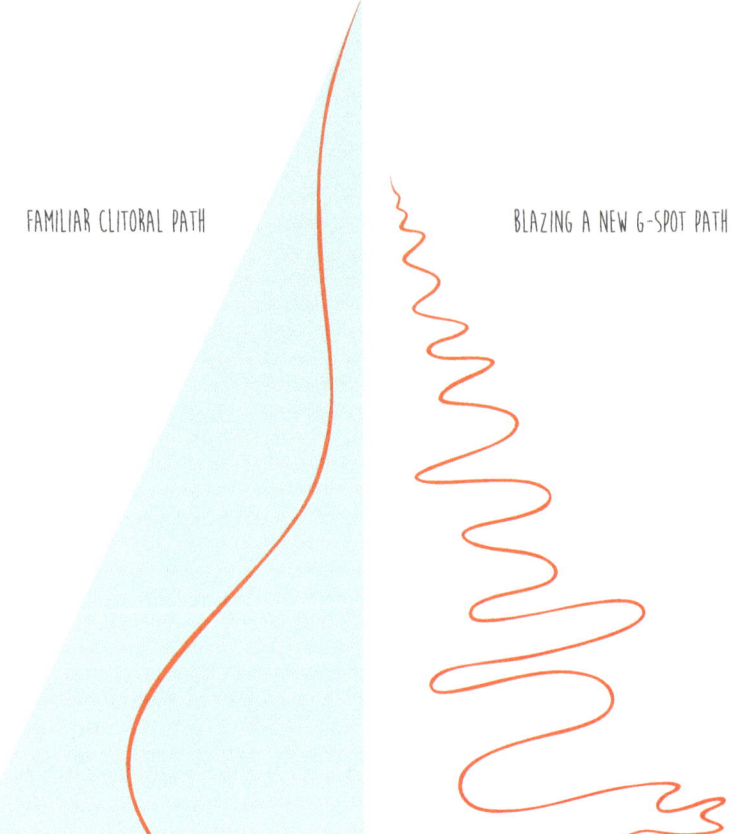

FAMILIAR CLITORAL PATH

BLAZING A NEW G-SPOT PATH

STRATEGY 2: CLIMB THE MOUNTAIN

Think of orgasm as a mountain. There are many ways to ascend the mountain, and each path looks and feels different. Most of us have followed roughly the same path—generally, the path of clitoral stimulation—for most of our lives. It's clear and well trodden, with familiar trees and bushes on either side. It's pretty easy to follow this path: some of us could even do it while asleep!

Climaxing from G-spot play, though, is like climbing that mountain via a completely different route. It requires a little more attention: noticing which way is up, fighting your way through thorny bushes, and being patient when the terrain isn't as easy or familiar. You may want to backtrack and return to that comfortable, familiar path—but you won't, because you're forging a new one. You're discovering different sensations

SWEET DREAMS

Skip the sleeping pills and the chamomile tea. Orgasm releases the hormones oxytocin and prolactin, which help you relax and fall asleep.

and erogenous areas that may have been hidden until now. And you're also becoming acclimatized to new patterns of arousal as you resist the temptation to scurry back to the safe path of clitoral stimulation. Ultimately, you may have to give your clitoris a rest for several—say, ten or twenty—pleasure sessions, until you've formed a new habit. (Horror! *Twenty* solo sex sessions *sans* clitoris? Now you know why this is the *second* recommended strategy.) This strategy helps you experience pleasure in a new way, without prejudice or expectation of what you think it is supposed to feel like. New erogenous zones will respond in new, unexpected ways, and it takes a bit of time to feel them out.

Once your body has learned a new way to climb the proverbial mountain, you'll be able to switch back and forth

MAKE MINE SWISS.

A 2011 survey on the C-Date dating site found that the Swiss are the most avid masturbators. A fine 92 percent of men and 72 percent of women engage in solo sex on a regular basis. More than 50 percent of women have used sex toys. And far from being threatened by them, almost one-third of Swiss men used sex toys with their partners.

between clitoral and G-spot play, or a combination of the two, anytime you like. And even if you couldn't find that second path up the mountain, you'll still have a better sense of what you like in terms of G-spot pleasure. And you can always return to—and celebrate—the amazing ways in which you're already able to come, because pleasure is fabulous, in all of its forms.

Now that your orgasmic potential is at its peak, it's time for a little fun *à deux*. But how do you translate solo sex orgasms to orgasms with a partner? Chapter 8 will show you how to make it happen.

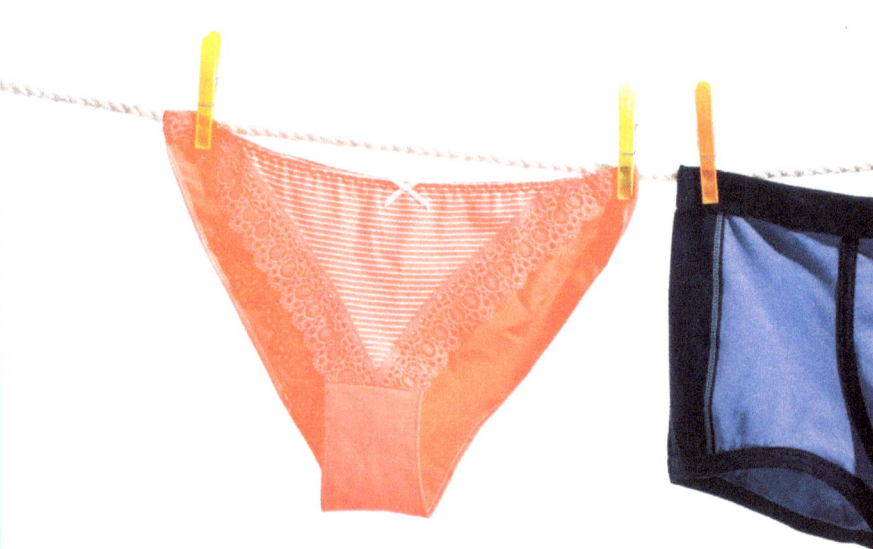
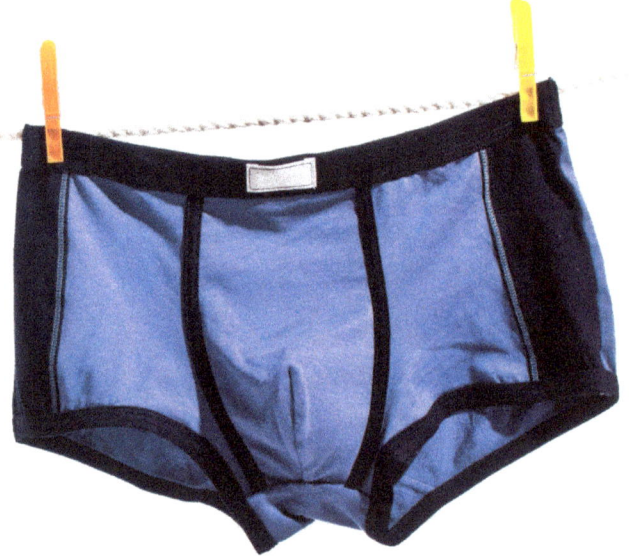

"MASTURBATION IS A DEMOCRATIC PLEASURE, PRACTICED BY RICH AND POOR, YOUNG AND OLD, MARRIED AND SINGLE."

Mason Cooley,
American aphorist

8 COMING TOGETHER

FROM ORGASMS ALONE TO ORGASMS WITH A PARTNER

As the old saying goes, two's company, right? Well, when it comes to orgasms, sometimes two can be a crowd. You'd think that coming during partner sex would be easier than it is when you're on your own, what with the extra excitement and intensity another person adds to the mix, but that's not necessarily so. Even if you can come quite quickly and easily while you're alone, it isn't always easy to translate your solo orgasms into orgasms during partner sex. Never fear, because this chapter will help you handle it. You'll find out why communication is the best sexual skill there is; how to open yourself to orgasming in front of, or even with, your partner; and how sex toys and games can make coming as a couple easier and more fun.

PARTNER SEX Q&A

HOW DO I START TALKING TO MY PARTNER ABOUT SOLO SEX?

It's great that you're ready to start sharing, because communication is the most effective erotic technique of all. Even if you and your partner are both spontaneous and love surprises, it's still important to talk to each other about your experiences and your desires. What have you learned about pleasure and your own body during your solo sex adventures? Would you like to incorporate some of it into your partnered sex life? What excites you about that, and what scares you? Of course, sometimes talking about sex is easier said than done. How do you initiate a conversation about partnered solo sex, especially if you haven't already been talking to each other about masturbation? How do you introduce your partner to new toys and techniques?

Some couples are very open with each other, and have no problem discussing their thoughts and feelings about sex. But lots of us find those conversations more than a little tricky. So, here's how to start talking about how to incorporate masturbation into your partnered sex life—and you might even find that these strategies can apply to other relationship issues, too.

First, bring up the topic casually, and don't do it while you're having sex. You might feel a little scared and vulnerable at first, but try to remember that frank, intimate conversations like these almost always bring both partners closer together. Second, clarify your intentions. What do you hope to achieve through this conversation? Perhaps you want to feel closer to your partner, to have better sex as a couple, or to add some variety to your sex life. Whatever your intentions are, be sure to articulate them to your partner. Third, be up front about your fears. Are you worried your partner will judge you or not be open to your suggestions? That you'll feel stupid even talking about sex? Tell them: It'll help your partner to listen with an open heart. Finally, use positive language, and emphasize how talking about solo sex can be great for your relationship. Tell your partner that exploration through masturbation is a fabulous way to improve partner sex, and that you want to share what you've learned. Explain that you've been trying to improve your sexual responses through solo sex, and that you want to integrate those responses into your shared sex life. Or simply say that you'd love to add partnered masturbation to your erotic repertoire.

A more playful (but no less informative) way to instigate a discussion about sex is to play a communication game called "Three Oranges and a Lemon." In it, each person tells the other three things that they love about their erotic life together, plus one thing that could be done differently. For example, you might say:

» "I love how you give me your full attention during oral sex until I come."

» "I love how you throw me up against the wall and kiss me deeply."

» "I love that you pleasure my whole body for a long time before touching my vulva."

» "And I'd love to try something different together—like masturbating in front of each other" (or using sex toys together, or playing out a masturbation fantasy: whatever it is you'd like to try).

It's okay to be a little less direct, if that's easier for you. Write out a masturbation fantasy that turns you on, then tell or show it to your partner (you can even email it to her, if you'd rather!). Then, pay attention to your partner's reaction: it might indicate whether or not he is willing to try it out. Or choose an erotic film that includes solo sex. Watch it together, and then ask your partner if she would like to see you do the same thing. Try a "fantasy share" as a couple: get your partner to write down five fantasies he would love to try out in real life, while you do the same. Include a fantasy or two that involves solo sex. When you're done, compare notes and

see which ideas appeal to both of you. (You might be surprised how similar your fantasies are!) Once you've broken the ice in these ways, try to ease your way into a candid conversation, because there's really no substitute for a straightforward discussion when it comes to sex—solo or otherwise.

HOW CAN MY PARTNER AND I COME TOGETHER?

If you're one of the many women who can orgasm alone but not with a partner, two is far from a magic number. But why is it so difficult to make the transition from orgasming alone to doing it *à deux*? There's no single answer to that question. A number of factors might be responsible. First of all, we're told that the act of masturbation is supposed to be "private." Even if you weren't shamed for touching yourself as a child, chances are a grownup told you firmly, "We do *that* in private." In this way, then, you were taught that self-pleasure is a solo activity that should have no witnesses, consenting or otherwise. What this means for you as an adult is, you feel embarrassed or self-conscious about coming when there's another person in the room. After all, if you're used to orgasming on your own, it makes sense that the idea of letting another person see and hear you might feel scary, intimidating, or embarrassing (except for exhibitionists, of course!). This reluctance to let go and allow another person into your experience of orgasm can hold you back from expressing your erotic self fully—and that makes orgasm less probable.

Emotional complications may be involved as well. If you've tried many times to come with your partner present but haven't had any success, then negative emotions may be standing in your way. Your partner might feel guilty that she or he can come while you can't. Or you may feel resentful of your partner's ability to enjoy pleasure so easily. While feelings like these are completely understandable, they're not

helpful: they can prevent you from relaxing and focusing on your own body. And speaking of relaxing, it's also true that most of us find it harder to relax while we're being watched—whether we're creating a work of art, solving a problem, or learning a new skill. So if your partner is a voyeur in the best sense of the word—someone who enjoys watching another person's arousal—it can be doubly hard to relax, because performance anxiety and pressure cancel out most of the fun.

Thirdly, you might feel that your partner's presence places pressure on you in a couple of different ways. For instance, that age-old question "Did you come?" generally kills the potential to come. Don't get me wrong, wanting to please your partner through having an orgasm in order to feel equal, fair, or closer together, or to share a special moment, is a worthy and righteous goal. But remember that pressure kills our arousal and orgasms. So when the

outcome of your performance dictates the tone of the relationship, the resulting pressure can negate all of these good intentions.

Then there's the fear of being judged or looking silly in front of your partner. Perhaps you worry that your partner might be turned off or disgusted by the technique you use to come, such as squeezing your legs together, or by what we look like as we self-pleasure. Because you probably don't know what you look like when you come, you might wonder: Is my face scrunched? Are my eyes shut? Is my mouth lopsided? Do the noises I make when I come sound sexy, or are they a huge turn-off? My naked body is exposed to my partner, and I feel so vulnerable; what if I don't look that attractive to her or him? These are just a few of the doubts that can plague you when you're trying to share your orgasm with a partner.

WHAT IF MY PARTNER GETS UPSET THAT I DON'T ORGASM?

Even when your partner has your best interests at heart, being unable to orgasm together can create tension and disappointment within a relationship. Your partner may feel inadequate, unskilled, and unattractive—not least because Hollywood movies would have us believe that all you need to do to bring your partner happiness and sexual fulfillment is to love him well. But that's grossly untrue. The fact is, inability to orgasm can and does occur within healthy, intensely loving, appreciative relationships. (And the opposite is also true: Sex can be satisfying and orgasmic even in relationships that aren't healthy at all!)

If your partner is frustrated because you can't orgasm as a couple, it might help to remind her or him that:

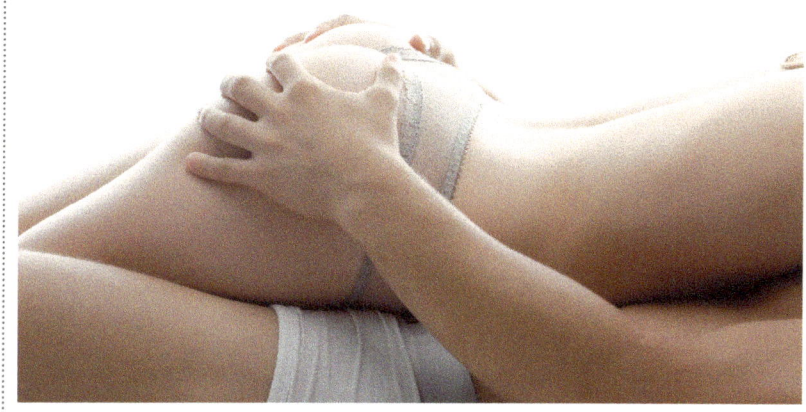

» IT'S ABOUT YOU. An orgasm is like a garden plant: You and your partner can plant a seed together and do everything you can to create an ideal environment for it, but whether the plant flourishes or not is out of your partner's control. Remind your partner that this is about you, not him, and that it'll happen when it happens.

» YOU CAN'T "GIVE" SOMEONE AN ORGASM. If and when an orgasm happens for you, your partner will be a lucky accomplice and witness to a beautiful, powerful event. Even if your partner is contributing formidable skill and lots of effort to encourage it, your orgasm is your own: no one can gift it to you.

» YOU STILL ENJOY THE PLEASURE. Tell your partner that you're attracted to her (and be specific!). What do you enjoy about the erotic time you spend

together? How does it bring you pleasure? Reassurance will help your partner feel more secure.

» PRESSURE KILLS. Explain to your partner that you love how important your pleasure is to her, but taking offense when you're not able to orgasm pressures you to prioritize the other person's feelings, not your own. And that can create even more distance between you and the amazing sensations that you're trying to enjoy as a couple.

» YOU DON'T WANT TO FAKE IT. Many women fake orgasms when they feel overwhelmed by the stress of not having an authentic one. Be honest with your partner, and tell him that you're not interested in faking it: You want to feel pleasure for real. And that'll happen when you're comfortable with the possibility of *not* coming.

HOW CAN I TRY TO HAVE AN ORGASM IN FRONT OF MY PARTNER?

If you can have an orgasm on your own, but not with your partner, try this: Pleasure yourself in exactly the same way that you do when you're flying solo—only do it with your partner present. While you're getting busy, she can watch you, kiss you, or touch you in ways that enhance the sensations—or he can pleasure himself at the same time. Consider asking your partner to talk to you in ways that turn you on: She might tell you how sexy you look, how much she loves you, or how exciting it is for her to watch you. Or, he could describe an erotic fantasy to you: It could be about an encounter you've already had, a fantasy you both share, or just about anything that gets you both going.

Still having trouble letting go? Try this technique again, and do it when your partner is in the room but is less engaged with what you're doing. For example, the two of you could sit or lie back-to-back—sometimes not facing each other takes the pressure off. Or your partner might be occupied with reading, watching TV, or another activity. You can also use a blindfold: Cover your partner's eyes, then pleasure yourself under the sheets, or blindfold yourself and then masturbate. (Adding a blindfold to the mix can be extra sexy, too, with its connotations of kink!)

If that's not working for you, see whether you can achieve orgasm if your partner is outside the room, or in another part of the house, or even down the street. Or try having phone sex—your partner can talk to you while you're doing it, if you like, or you ask her to just listen. Once you've had an orgasm, you can try again, bringing your partner a little closer to you physically each time.

A few other techniques can be helpful. Ask your partner to pleasure *himself* while you watch; afterward, discuss the experience and your feelings about it. When the shoe is on the other foot, you might realize that watching can be arousing—and if you're not judging your partner when she pleasures herself, it's likely that she isn't judging you either. Another way to normalize the experience is to just do it, without a lot of fanfare. Don't announce your intention; just reach down and start pleasuring yourself when you're kissing, having sex, or even just watching TV on the couch. Or if you'd rather, do the exact opposite: Turn the encounter into a performance instead! Start with a striptease or a lap dance; put on music, if you want to, and take control of the event. Tell your partner what she is and isn't allowed to do as she watches you. Go ahead and be playful: Get your partner to play the "voyeur" game, in which he stays quietly hidden behind the bedroom or closet door, peeking out to watch you self-pleasure. Tell him that he isn't allowed to come out until you say so; that way, you'll feel completely in control.

There are a few techniques you can try during partner sex, too. Start by touching yourself regularly during sex. Don't worry, you don't have to do it for a long time. Even touching yourself briefly during sex with your partner will make it feel more natural the next time. Or if you usually grind against your hand or a pillow to come during solo sex, then grind against your partner's hand, thigh, or side instead. If you don't often use a vibrator or massager during solo sex, try it with a partner. Small changes like these can make orgasm more likely.

Finally, when you're having solo sex, fantasize about doing it front of your partner. Make the fantasy hot and exciting, and imagine what your partner might do or want to do as she watches. If any self-judgmental thoughts creep into your head, repeat your mantra to yourself to help you replace those negative ideas with positive ones. And, don't forget to revisit chapter 6's ideas for enhancing pleasure, as well as chapter 7's ways to encourage an orgasm that's just out of reach.

It's so important to talk about your experiences after you try any of these techniques. Giving voice to your fears, reservations, or feelings of self-consciousness can go a long way toward alleviating them. Hearing about your partner's experience is equally helpful: He'll be able to tell you how much he enjoys watching you, how hot you look, and how it turns him on. Plus, your partner can act as your mirror, reflecting habits you might not be able to notice on your own. For instance, she might notice that you tend to tense up or stop breathing, or that you're focusing on something other than pleasure. This feedback can help you break free from unproductive patterns, and to learn and grow.

I CAN BRING MYSELF TO ORGASM IN FRONT OF MY PARTNER, BUT MY PARTNER CAN'T DO IT FOR ME. CAN I CHANGE THAT?

It's wonderful that you and your partner can orgasm together! But wouldn't it be great if your partner could bring you there on his own? If that's not possible for you right now, it may be due to an excessive focus on intercourse as *the* way of achieving orgasm. Remember that only 30 percent of women can orgasm during intercourse without clitoral stimulation, while another 19 percent can get there as long as clitoral stimulation is also involved. So if you can't push yourself over the edge—or even feel much pleasure—from vaginal stimulation alone, try to let go of those expectations. Forcing yourself to orgasm in a certain way is unreasonable, especially when there are so many ways to do it!

Even if your partner is doing exactly what you do when you are going solo, he doesn't have the immediate feedback from your hands to your erogenous zones and back to your brain that you have when you touch yourself. Thus, it makes sense that your partner's technique is not as effective and responsive as yours is. Like the game of broken telephone, we have to be really clear and sometimes reframe and repeat what we need in order to have it translate into the pleasure that works for us.

Here are some ways to bring your partner into your solo sex adventures.

» **EXPERIMENT WITH A NEW WAY TO COME.** Remember the two techniques in chapter 7 for learning a new way to orgasm? Here's the partnered version: Touch yourself until you're close to the edge, and finish off the deed with your partner's touch. Or, for a predetermined length of time, stop touching yourself during solo and/or partner sex, and try "reprogramming" your erotic response with the new sensations your partner offers.

» **BE HANDS-ON.** Place your hand over your partner's to show him what you like in terms of rhythm, pressure, length, and speed of stroke, and when to increase or decrease the level of intensity.

» **GIVE FEEDBACK.** Talk about what works and what doesn't, and be as specific as possible. Tell your partner what she's doing right, and what you'd like her to modify. For example, you might say, "I love that level of speed, but could you go a little more gently?" Specific feedback will help your partner understand exactly what you want and how you want it.

» **DON'T GIVE UP.** The classic frustration is that you ask for it more gently (say, a 3 on a scale of 1 to 10 of pressure). Your partner was at an 8 and reduces the pressure to a 6. Don't give up. Recognize that your partner is trying but needs a little more direction. You can use the scale to help her understand the pressure, or you can acknowledge her effort and reframe your request as: "That IS more gently, can you do it even gentler *still*, please."

» **GET CREATIVE.** Depending on your individual interests, try lots of different sexual techniques: oral sex; pleasure via fingers, toys, or breasts; intercourse; anal sex; kink; dominance and submission; bondage; fantasy; or just about anything else that turns you on.

» **WRITE YOUR OWN STORY.** Imagine an ideal sex scene between you and your partner, and then write it down—and don't leave anything out. Be explicit about what you're doing, when you're doing it, and how. Emphasize what's important to you, and the type of emotional connection you want: is it hot, sensual, adventurous, tender, wild, or healing? Then show your story to your partner. The more detail you use, the better, because that'll help your partner understand what works for you.

WHAT IF MY PARTNER FEELS THREATENED BY USING A SEX TOY?

Lots of women only use sex toys on their own, usually because they're afraid of bruising their partners' egos, or because playing with a toy simply feels like a "private" activity. But many lovers of women (of both genders) really enjoy using toys as a couple. And the best way to convince your partner that a toy can be fun is to try it on her! Blindfold your partner first, if you like, to limit any expectations about what the toy is "supposed to do." Then, practice the techniques you learned in chapter 5 for using toys with a partner (see page 101). The more your partner feels that the sex toy's role is to pleasure *both* of you, regardless of gender, the more open to it he will be. You could even get your partner a toy of her own so that you can each use them on yourselves at the same time. In this way, toys become a shared experience and a way to expand the possibilities of partner sex.

If your partner still feels threatened by a sex toy, please reassure her or him that the toy is an enhancement of your relationship, not a replacement for it. Remind her that you find her attractive,

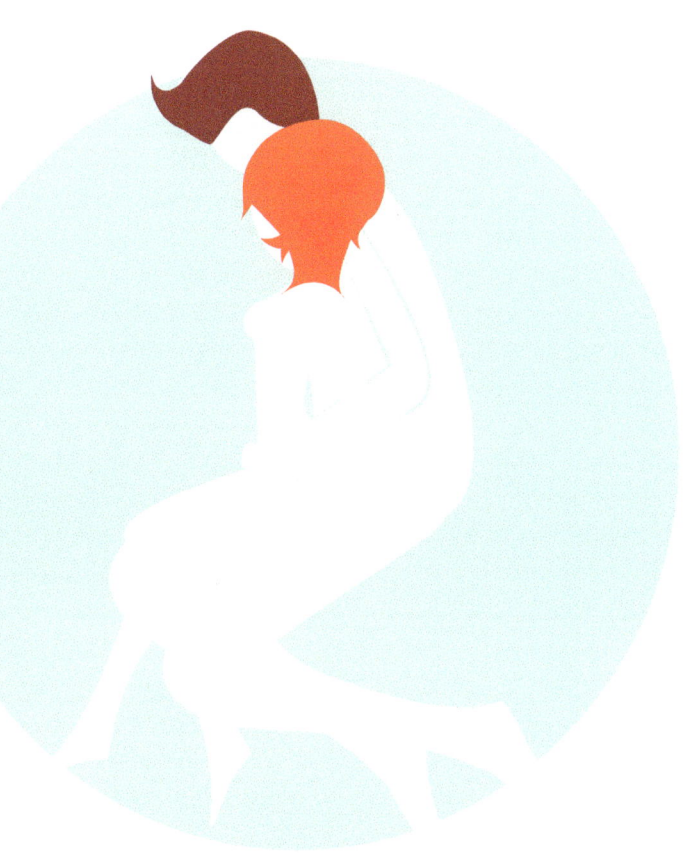

and tell her why. Point out that using a toy can make his job way easier, especially if bringing you to orgasm takes a lot of effort. Emphasize the fact that a toy can add some variety to your sex romps, and tell her it's like having a few extra hands to help with the work! Ultimately, a toy can never compete with a person. You'll never leave a real, live partner for a vibrator: A vibrator won't take you out for a great night on the town; it doesn't respond when you lick or suck it; and it can't pleasure your entire body in ways that your partner's warm, versatile hands can.

Do give your partner some space and time without pressure to try any kind of sex, including solo sex together and using toys together. There are no rules that govern what you "should" or "should not" do together, and sometimes a partner needs a little time to reflect before coming around to the idea. She or he might find it helpful to talk to friends, or to do some Internet research on what other couples do. After a few chats (or clicks), it's likely that your partner will conclude that it's very common for couples to bring masturbation or sex toys into partner sex. But nobody likes to be shamed or forced into accepting a new idea—especially when it comes to sex!—so give your partner some time before carefully and lovingly broaching the subject again.

You may feel self-conscious about bringing a sex toy that you've only used for solo play into your relationship: It can be a little like inviting an old lover to join the two of you! That's okay. If you don't feel ready to share your solo toy, you can buy a new one together. It's a great opportunity to upgrade, and to get a toy that's even better than the one you already have in terms of size, power, versatility, quality, or function. Or get something that appeals to both of you and can be used in ways that delight each of you, making sex better for both.

SOLO SEX GAMES FOR TWO

Sure, you can enjoy solo sex with your partner when you're both feeling erotic. But the great thing about masturbation is that it's not necessary for both of you to be in the mood at the same time. Even if you or your partner isn't up for full sex at the moment, you can still be a part of each other's solo experience—without forcing yourself to get aroused or having sex when you don't really want to. And being the more passive participant in a partnered solo sex encounter can be a lot of fun! You might whisper a fantasy in your partner's ear, kiss her mouth or cover her entire body with kisses, massage his scalp, or touch her in any way she enjoys. Or you could simply watch appreciatively. (There's just one drawback to this technique, though: It tends to put the less-horny person in the mood for sex! If that happens, you can just reverse the roles after your partner is finished—or you can turn the experience into a pleasure adventure for two.)

That's where the following scenarios come in. These erotic games are a fun way to kick off your next partnered solo sex romp. Of course, you should feel free to modify them in any way that arouses you, and you can switch up the roles as well. Go ahead and make them your own!

LONG-DISTANCE LOVE

HOW DO WE PLAY? Whether your partner is in the next room, at work in the next city, or on the other side of the world, you can call her and pleasure yourself while on the phone with her. Ask your partner to tell you about his favorite fantasy, have him relive the best sex you've ever had together, or get him to tell you what he's going to do to you the next time he sees you. If you'd rather be the storyteller, that's fine—but you'll probably be out of breath before you can finish!

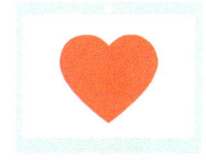

VARIATIONS: Tell your partner that she's not allowed to touch herself during the call, or until the next time you see each other. Make him wait for you—your next encounter will be that much hotter. Or get her to pleasure herself, too—with the caveat that she has to do what you tell her, then describe how it feels. You can also add a little role-play, if you like. Who do you want to be today? A movie star? A character from a novel? A sexy stranger? Take it to the next level by playing out a scene, such as a naughty housewife and a pushy door-to-door salesperson who is prepared to do anything to secure the next sale.

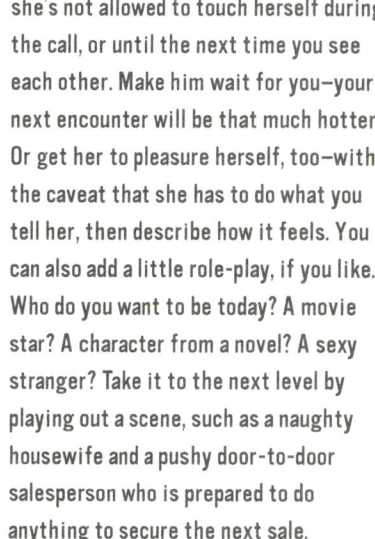

THE EXHIBITIONIST AND THE VOYEUR

HOW DO WE PLAY? Dress up in clothes that make you feel sexy, whether it's leather, lace, office attire, or beachwear. Have your partner sit in a chair while you lie on the bed or couch. Pretend that you're a stripper at a club and you're trying to get a good tip. Work hard for your money—but don't work it too fast. Take your time and tease your partner and yourself.

VARIATIONS: Come up with a few different outfits, and lay them out on the bed, couch, or kitchen table for your partner. Get him to choose your attire and accoutrements for the sex session (or ask him to help you pick out something new for the occasion). Or get in touch with your inner dominatrix, and tell your partner what she is and isn't allowed to do. Perhaps she's not allowed to touch herself—or maybe she has to touch herself in the way you want her to. Imagine what the strip club looks like, and get her to describe it to you in detail. Move around so that your partner gets a good look at different parts of your body: your face, butt, vulva, legs, breasts. Place a mirror in the room, and angle it so that your partner can see your reflection, too.

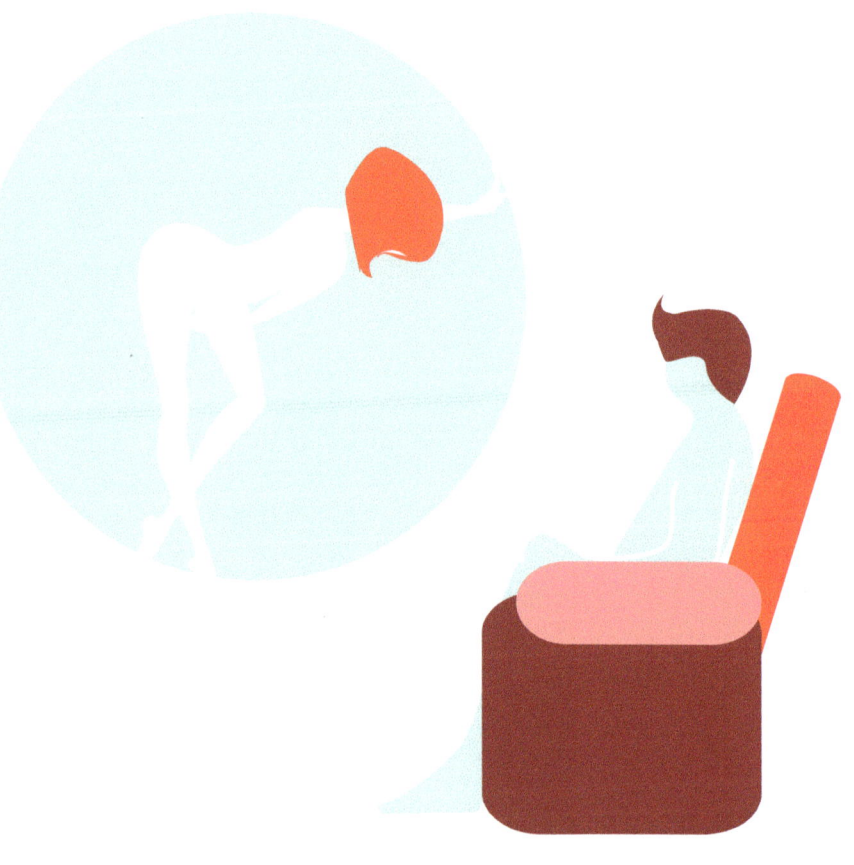

THE LUXURIOUS LAP DANCE

HOW DO WE PLAY? Seat your partner in a comfortable chair, and give her the lap dance of her dreams. Ride his thighs and hips for your own pleasure. You can use your hands or a toy to stroke yourself, but tell your partner that she isn't allowed to touch you—or herself—at all. (That's a guaranteed turn-on!) Take your clothes off slowly, piece by piece, and touch yourself as you work. Rub yourself against his clothed body, and watch him drool.

VARIATIONS: Touching is against the rules! If your partner breaks those rules, she'll have to be "punished." Threaten to tie him to the chair so he'll have no choice but to behave. Then, make good on that threat: Grab some nylon rope, and gently but firmly tie her down so she can see that you mean business. Or place a sex toy against his leg or crotch, and grind against it solely for your own pleasure. Tell her what it would be like to have sex with her right then and there. Blindfold him, and tell him you'll stop what you're doing if he dares to peek. Then keep moving around her, letting her feel your touch and presence more intensely now that one of her senses has been restrained.

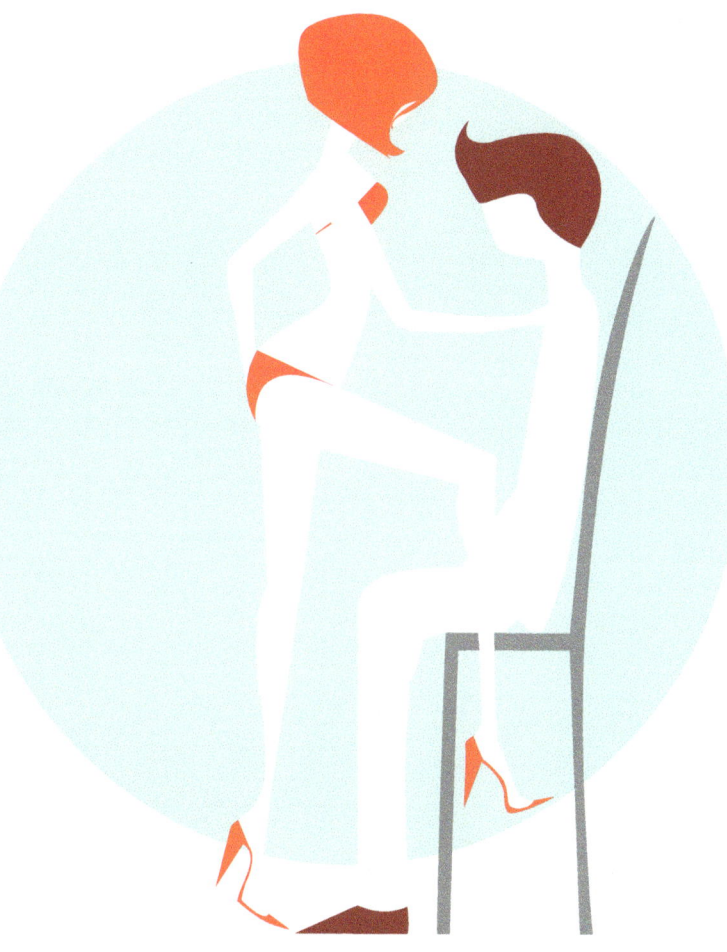

SHOW AND TELL

HOW DO WE PLAY? Try this variation of "I'll show you mine if you show me yours." Pretend the two of you are strangers, or even inexperienced teenagers, if you like. Take turns showing each other your erogenous zones and how you like to be touched. Incorporate toys, lube, and anything else that turns you on, such as your favorite fantasies. The partner who's watching can ask questions and observe like a good student, or she can simply sit back and appreciate the show. The whole experience can feel like a fantasy, an educational experience, or even both!

VARIATIONS: Be an active observer. While your partner's showing you what he likes, describe his actions out loud so you'll be better able to remember them for next time. When it's your turn, do the same thing. Explaining what you're doing helps your partner focus, and makes the entire experience hotter. Tell your partner what you want him to think about while you're doing the showing: giving you oral sex, imagining that you're outdoors, or indulging in sex play in a public place, or that you're the first woman he's ever been with. Or film your show-and-tell session. (Just make sure you come to an agreement on where the file should be stored, and whether or when it should be destroyed.)

FIFTY SHADES OF "DO AS I SAY"

HOW DO WE PLAY? In this game, one partner assumes a dominant role, and issues sexy instructions to the other. The dominant partner can be polite ("Please take off your clothes"), directive ("Take off your clothes"), seductive ("I'd love to watch you take off your clothes for me"), suggestive ("If you take off your clothes, I'll give you some fun toys to play with"), or can act in any way that feels good to both of you.

VARIATIONS: Get permission from your dominant partner before you're allowed to orgasm. Are you allowed to have multiple orgasms, or do you have to stop at just one? Or your partner might direct you until you're on the brink of an orgasm, and then tell you to stop. Your partner might pleasure himself and/or touch your body while giving directions. Add extra excitement by adding (gentle) physical constraints: Being unable to move your arms and legs makes orgasm a fun challenge.

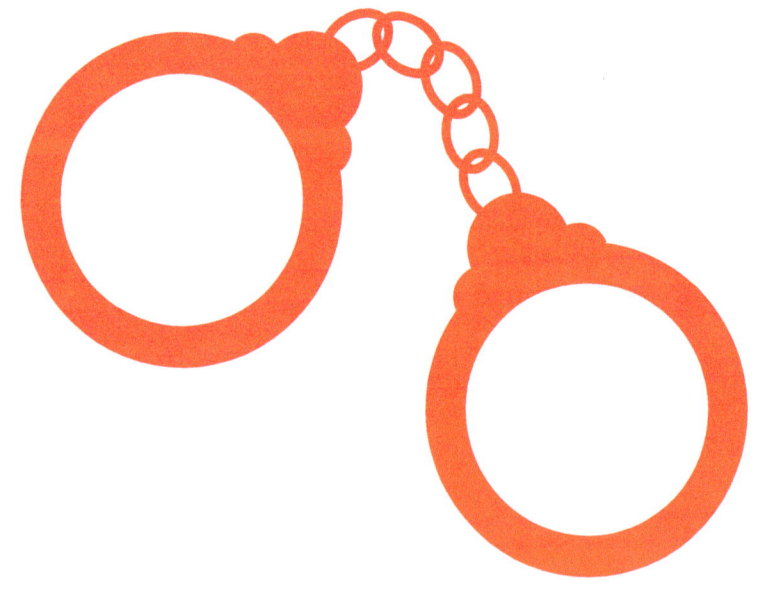

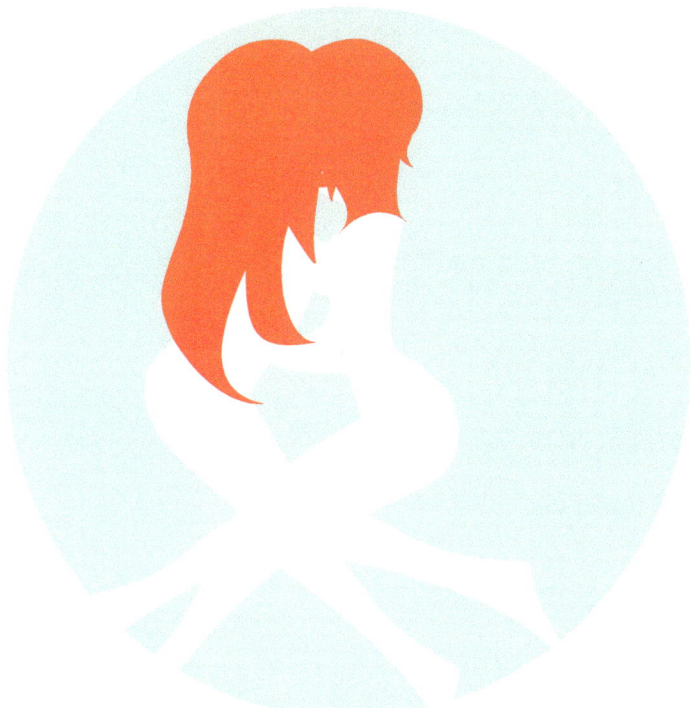

THE WINDOWS TO THE SOUL

HOW DO WE PLAY? Lie down side by side or sit facing each other, looking into each other's eyes. Then, each of you can pleasure yourself—but don't break eye contact throughout the sex session. That makes for an incredibly intense and intimate experience. (It's not about staring each other down, though: Some people find it easier to maintain contact by focusing on the spot between their partner's eyebrows. If you're finding it really difficult to maintain eye contact, do take breaks by looking away for a moment, or closing your eyes.)

VARIATIONS: Kiss each other on the lips while maintaining eye contact. It's a little more challenging, but it's worth it: Having a point of physical contact with one another during solo sex really ramps up the pleasure. Try breathing in tandem, or in opposite patterns (that is, one of you breathes in while the other breathes out). Talk to each other: Fantasize out loud about where you might be or what you might be doing. Or simply talk about what turns you on. Rub against each other as you pleasure yourselves. Tell your partner what you'd like to see him do. And remember, intense and intimate doesn't necessarily have to be serious: Make it fun!

NAKED MIME

HOW DO WE PLAY? Lie down side by side or stand up facing one other. Nominate one person to be the "leader," while the other is the "follower" (take turns so that you both get to experience each role). If you're the follower for now, watch the leader masturbate, and imitate his movements: If you're differently gendered, you can still replicate your partner's moves, just imitate the stroke in a way that makes sense in the context of your own body. Then switch roles.

VARIATIONS: Try to time your orgasms so that you both come at the same time. Do it side by side, both of you looking in the mirror in front of you. Grab a toy each, and try to imitate what your partner is doing with his or hers. Try a move that's challenging for the other person to imitate—that'll force her to be creative. (This game might have you both doubled up with laughter instead of pleasure, but that's totally fine, and it's part of the fun! Just refocus, then try again or shift to another style of play.)

CONCLUSION

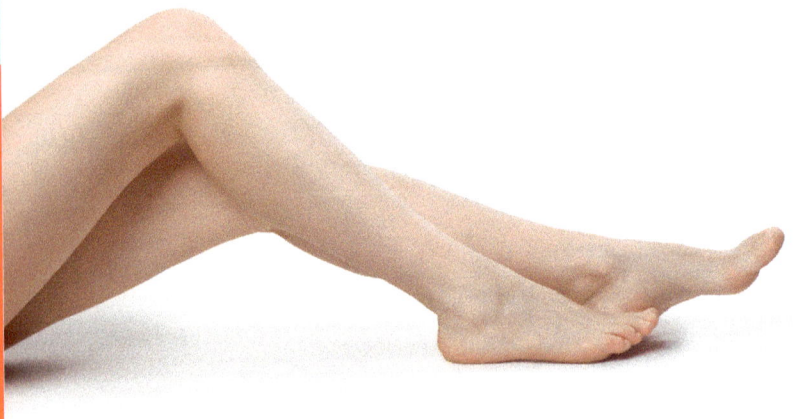

Hopefully, this book has helped you explore and appreciate your body's beauty and its potential for pleasure. And perhaps it's led you to address assumptions or reservations about sex and sexuality that may have held you back from experimenting with solo sex. It might even have taught you a few (or more than a few!) new skills and techniques to boot. Here are a few parting words that I hope you'll remember as you embark on brand-new solo sex adventures.

YOUR BODY IS BEAUTIFUL, AND PLEASURE IS YOUR BIRTHRIGHT. Whatever shape, size, age, and ability level you are, know that your body is awesome. If popular media has influenced your attitude toward your body by imposing conventional, two-dimensional, unrealistic standards upon it, then it's up to you to actively reject those standards. Connect with others who are creating new versions and visions of what "beautiful" is. You can choose to be your own best advocate—and your own best friend—by embracing and celebrating your body's distinctive qualities. Know that pleasure is good, whether it comes from delicious food, gorgeous scenery, beautiful music, seductive smells, or delightful physical sensations. Taking pleasure in your own body is a healthy, honorable, and important task. It's good for your physical health, emotional well-being, and self-esteem, and the confidence you develop as a result can only enhance your erotic relationships.

THERE IS NO "RIGHT WAY." Just as your body is unique, so are its desires, erogenous zones, and responses. What works for your best friend might not work for you—and that's fine. So go ahead and develop your own recipes for pleasure! As long as you're not harming yourself or others, the options for pleasure are endless. Open your mind to the people and situations you find sexy, either in your fantasies or in real life. Think about exploring different kinds of sex—from romantic to kinky, solo to multiple-partnered, fingers to penises to vaginas to toys. Life is about trying things on for size to see how they fit, so experiment within your own boundaries, and allow your erotic identity to unfold in all its glory.

THE JOURNEY IS THE DESTINATION. Enjoy each step in the process of arousal, from conjuring up sexy fantasies to the subtle (or intense!) sensations that solo sex offers to the orgasms that happen en route. Remember that orgasm is only *one* step in the journey, so don't make it the entire focus. After all, pressuring yourself to "get there" will only make you less likely to enjoy the full experience, and what's more, it'll make you less likely to orgasm at all. Performance levels and goals may feature in your office life, but try to banish them from your sex life.

MAKE THE MOST OF IT. This journey is yours for the taking: no one else can take it for you. It's up to you to value your sexual growth and revel in your glorious body and its wonders. Yes, life is all about balancing priorities, and you've got your career, family and community, personal development, and healthy lifestyle to consider. But your sexual health is just as important, and the good news is, nurturing it only takes a few minutes per day or a few hours per week. And its benefits are immense. So indulge in a lifetime of pleasure—and enjoy!

RESOURCES

DVDS

Anal Massage for Relaxation and Pleasure, directed by Joseph Kramer, Ph.D. Endless anal play, either alone or with a partner.

—

Female Ejaculation for Couples, directed by Deborah Sundahl. Great for both couples and individuals, this DVD explains what female ejaculation is and where it comes from.

—

Red Hot Touch: Genital Massage for Women, directed by New World Sex Education. This DVD illustrates lots of different strokes; it's ideal for either solo or partnered pleasure.

—

Tristan Taormino's Expert Guide to the G-Spot, directed by Tristan Taormino. Sex educator and award-winning director Taormino's DVD shows you everything you need to know about the G-spot: where it is, how to find it, which toys can help you pleasure it, and lots more.

BOOKS

The Elusive Orgasm: A Woman's Guide to Why She Can't and How She Can Orgasm by Vivienne Cass. Learn how to orgasm or how to come more consistently during solo or partnered sex.

—

Female Ejaculation and the G-spot by Deborah Sundahl. Detailed information about the G-spot, including how to find it and how to ejaculate.

—

The Guide to Getting it On by Paul Joannides, PsyD. A straightforward guide to sex and pleasure.

—

Healing Sex: A Mind-Body Approach to Healing Sexual Trauma by Staci Haines. Information plus a workbook to help you find pleasure in sex after experiencing trauma.

—

I Love Female Orgasm by Dorian Solot and Marshall Miller. An in-depth guide to female orgasm for women and their partners.

—

I'll Show You Mine by Wrenna Robertson. Diverse images of unique vulvas.

—

The Little Book of Kink: Sexy Secrets for Thrilling Over-the-Edge Pleasure by Jessica O'Reilly, Ph.D. Easy suggestions for bringing a little kink into your sex life.

—

Love in the Time of Colic: The New Parents Guide to Getting It on Again by Ian Kerner, Ph.D., and Heidi Raykei. Strategies to help new parents find time, desire, and energy for sex.

—

Naked at Our Age: Talking Out Loud about Senior Sex by Joan Price. Seniors get it on, too! Here's how to make senior sex even better.

—

Orgasm: Photographs and Interviews by Linda Troeller and Marion Schneider. Diverse images of women experiencing orgasm, plus their personal narratives.

—

Reclaiming Desire: 4 Keys to Finding Your Lost Libido by Andrew Goldstein, M.D., and Marianne Brandon, Ph.D. Learn how to boost your libido and develop more desire for sex.

—

Secrets of the Sex Masters by Carl Frankel. Tips on making sex, solo or partnered, even better.

—

Sex for One by Betty Dodson. The classic book on becoming comfortable with self-pleasure.

Sex Recharge: A Rejuvenation Plan for Couples and Singles by Ian Kerner, Ph.D. A detailed workbook on (re)discovering pleasure and creating the erotic life of your dreams.

—

Slow Sex: The Art and Craft of the Female Orgasm by Nicole Daedone. A partner program for receiving pleasure and enjoying non-orgasm-focused sex.

—

Urban Tantra: Sacred Sex for the Twenty-First Century by Barbara Carrellas. Tantric sex for everyone, regardless of sexual orientation or religious affiliation.

—

When Sex Hurts by Andrew Goldstein, M.D., and Caroline Pukall, M.D. Goldstein and Pukall show you how to pinpoint the source and type of pain, and offer suggestions for pelvic pain management.

—

The Whole Lesbian Sex Book: A Passionate Guide for All of Us by Felice Newman. A comprehensive guide to culture, terminology, and sexual practices between women.

—

Women's Anatomy of Arousal by Sheri Winston, C.N.M., R.N., B.S.N., L.M.T. Detailed, easy-to-understand information on our erotic anatomy, and how to enjoy more pleasure during arousal and sex.

WEBSITES

The Adipositivity Project (www.adipositivity.com): Images of people of all sizes, clothed and naked.

—

Disabled People are Sexy (www.tumview.com/disabledpeoplearesexy): Celebrating the sexiness of people with disabilities.

—

The Scar Project (www.thescarproject.org): Women sharing their beauty and the scars they carry as a result of breast cancer.

WHERE TO BUY

USA

Albuquerque, NM: Self Serve (www.selfservetoys.com)

—

Baltimore, MD: Sugar (www.sugartheshop.com)

—

Chicago, IL: Early to Bed (www.early2bedshop.com)

—

Milwaukee, WI: The Tool Shed (www.toolshedtoys.com)

—

Minneapolis, MN: Smitten Kitten (www.smittenkittenonline.com)

—

Northampton, MA: Oh My (www.ohmysensuality.com)

—

Oakland, CA: Feelmore 510 (www.Feelmore510.com)

—

Portland, ME: Nomia (www.nomiaboutique.com)

—

Portland, OR: She Bop (www.sheboptheshop.com)

CANADA

Ottawa, ON, and Halifax, NS: Venus Envy (www.venusenvy.ca)

—

Richmond Hill, ON: Dick and Jane Romance Boutique (www.dickandjane.ca)

—

Toronto, ON: Good For Her (www.goodforher.com)

UK

Edinburgh: Q Store

—

London: Sh! (www.sh-womenstore.com)

REFERENCES

INTRODUCTION

Herbenick, D., and J. D. Fortenberry. 2011. "Exercise-induced orgasm and pleasure among women." *Sexual and Relationship Therapy* 26 (4): 373–88.

Laumann, E., J. Gagnon, R. Michael, and S. Michaels. 1994. *The Social Organization of Sexuality: Sexual Practices in the United States*. Chicago: University of Chicago Press.

CHAPTER 1

LoPiccolo, J. and W.E. Stock. 1986. "Treatment of sexual dysfunction." *Journal of Consulting and Clinical Psychology* 54 (2), 158–67.

Hurlbert, D., and K. E. Whittaker. 1991. "The role of masturbation in marital and sexual satisfaction: a comparative study of female masturbators and nonmasturbators." *Journal of Sex Education and Therapy* 17 (4): 272–82.

Michael, R. T., J. H. Gagnon, E. O. Laumann, and G. Kolata. 1994. *Sex in America: A Definitive Survey*. Boston: Little, Brown and Company.

Gerressu, M., C. H. Mercer, C. A. Graham, K. Wellings, and A. M. Johnson. 2008. "Prevalence of masturbation and associated factors in a British national probability survey." *Archive of Sexual Behaviour* 37 (2): 266–78.

Shulman, J. L., and S. G. Horne. 2003. "The use of self-pleasure: masturbation and body image among African American and European American women." *Psychology of Women Quarterly* 27 (3): 262–69.

Anderson, T., V. Schick, D. Herbenick, B. Dodge, J. Fortenberry. 2014. "A study of human papillomavirus on vaginally inserted sex toys, before and after cleaning, among women who have sex with women and men." *Sexually Transmitted Infections* 2014 (0): 1–3.

Hogarth, H., and R. Ingham. 2009. "Masturbation among young women and associations with sexual health: an exploratory study. *The Journal of Sex Research* 46 (6): 558–67.

Crooks, R., and K. Baur. 1983. "Sexual behavior patterns." *In Our Sexuality*. Menlo Park, CA: The Benjamin/Cummings Publishing Company.

Stein, Daniel S. 1999. *Passionate Sex*. New York: Carroll & Graf Publishers.

Brody, Stuart. 2004. "Slimness is associated with greater intercourse and less masturbation frequency." *Journal of Sex and Marital Therapy* 30 (4): 251–61.

Mamtani, M. R., and H. R. Kulkarni. 2005. "Predictive performance of anthropometric indexes of central obesity for the risk of type-2 diabetes." *Archives of Medical Research* 36 (5): 581–89.

Rexrode, K. M., V. J. Carey, C. H. Hennekens, et al. 1998. "Abdominal adiposity and coronary heart disease in women." *Journal of the American Medical Association* 280 (21):1843–48.

Smith, D. A., et al. 2005. "Abdominal diameter index: a more powerful anthropometric measure for prevalent coronary heart disease risk in adult males." *Diabetes Obesity Metabolism* 7 (4): 370–80.

Costa, R. M., and S. Brody. 2012. "Greater resting heart rate variability is associated with orgasms through penile-vaginal intercourse, but not with orgasms from other sources." *Journal of Sexual Medicine* 9 (1): 188–97.

Komisaruk, B., and B. Whipple. 1995. "The suppression of pain by genital stimulation in females." *Annual Review of Sex Research* 6 (1): 151–86.

Cooper, S. C., and A. Santella. 2013. "Happy news! Masturbation actually has health benefits." http://theconversation.com/happy-news-masturbation-actually-has-health-benefits-16539.

Glasper, E. R., and E. Gould. 2013. "Sexual experience restores age-related decline in adult neurogenesis and hippocampal function." *Hippocampus* 23 (4): 303–12.

Lopiccolo and Lobitiz, 1972.

Hambach, A., S. Evers, O. Summ, I. Hussedt, and A. Frese. 2013. "The impact of sexual activity on idiopathic headaches: an observational study." *Cephalagia* 33 (6): 384–89.

Brody, Stuart. 2006. "Blood pressure reactivity to stress is better for people who recently had penile–vaginal intercourse than for people who had other or no sexual activity." *Biological Psychology* 71 (2): 214–22.

Whipple, B., and B. Komisaruk. 1988. "Analgesia produced in women by genital self-stimulation." *The Journal of Sex Research* 24 (1): 130–40.

Kim, J. I., J. W. Lee, Y. A. Lee, D. H. Lee, N. S. Han, Y. K. Choi, et al. 2013. "Sexual activity counteracts the suppressive effects of chronic stress on adult hippocampal neurogenesis and recognition memory." *Brain Research* 1538: 26–40.

Charnetski, C., and F. Brennan. 2004. "Sexual frequency and salivary immunoglobulin A (IGA)." *Psychological Reports* 94 (3): 839–44.

CHAPTER 2

Herbenick, D., M. Reece, V. S. A. Sanders, B. Dodge, and J. D. Fortenberry. 2010. "Sexual behavior in the United States: results from a national probability sample of men and women ages 14–94." *The Journal of Sexual Medicine* 7 (S5): 255–65.

CHAPTER 4

Kinsey, Alfred C., et al. *Sexual Behavior in the Human Female*. Philadelphia: W. B. Saunders; Bloomington, IN: Indiana U. Press, 1953/1998.

Santamaria, F. C. 1997. "Female Ejaculation, Myth and Reality." Presented at the Proceedings of 13th World Congress of Sexology, Valencia, Spain.

CHAPTER 6

Critelli, J., and J. Bivona. 2008. "Women's erotic rape fantasies: an evaluation of theory and research." *The Journal of Sex Research* 45 (1): 57–70.

CHAPTER 7.

Masters, W. H., and V. E. Johnson. 1966. *Human Sexual Response*. New York: Bantam Books.

Komisaruk, B. R., B. Whipple, A. Crawford, S. Grimes, W. C. Liu, A. Kalnin, et al. 2004. "Brain activation during vaginocervical self-stimulation and orgasm in women with complete spinal cord injury: fMRI evidence of mediation by the vagus nerves." *Brain Research* 1024 (1–2): 77–78.

De Sutter, P., J. Day, and F. Adam. 2014. "Who are the orgasmic women? Exploratory study among a community sample of French-speaking women." *Sexologies* 23 (3): e51–e57.

ABOUT THE AUTHOR

Carlyle Jansen is the founder of Good For Her, Toronto's premiere sexuality shop and workshop center, and producer of the annual Feminist Porn Awards. Popular for her straightforward approach, friendly humor, and down-to-earth disposition, she is a regular speaker at the Guelph Sex Therapy Training Program. Carlyle has also been teaching workshops , speaking at conferences and coaching individuals and couples looking to enhance their sexual lives since 1995. She's passionate about education for everyone, and her teaching audience ranges from sexual health professionals to youth and parents to university classes to gatherings in living rooms. She is a regular contributor to local print, radio, and television media, with appearances in many documentaries. Her chapter on sensational oral sex appears in the book *Secrets of the Sex Masters*. Follow her on Twitter @CarlyleJansen and find her other work at www.carlylejansen.com.

ACKNOWLEDGMENTS

Many thanks to my mom, who always encouraged me to follow my passions, even when she did not understand my enthusiasm for sexual education. I have much gratitude to my many teachers over the years, in particular all of those who have attended my workshops and private sessions. I could not have amassed what I know without your earnest questions about sex, stories of inspiration and challenge, and deep desire to create the sex lives that you deserve.

INDEX

A

abdomen, 31
ability levels, 47–48
age, 47
alcohol, 57, 66, 134
aloe vera, 68
ambiance, 118–119
Amorino, 104
anal techniques, 85–87
anterior fornix, 35
antidepressants, 132
antihistamines, 66
anti-masturbation products, 19
anus, 34
aphrodisiacs, 51–52
armpit, 30
Around the Clock Pleasure
  technique, 77
arousal, 58–59, 129, 134, 139
A-spot, 35, 82

B

back, 30
back massagers, 92
bacteria, 38, 87, 111
bathtub faucets, 91
birth control pill, 132
body
  exploration of, 131
  loving your, 45–49
body changes
  in menopause, 40–41
  post-pregnancy, 40
  in pregnancy, 38
  in puberty, 37
body image, 18, 20, 133

body massagers, 92
boredom, 139
breast-feeding, 40, 66, 133, 136
breasts, 30
breathing, 57, 120, 137
Bulb Massage technique, 72
butt, 31
butt plugs, 86, 107, 122

C

calves, 31
Captain's Chair, 87
carrageenan, 68
cell phones, 92
cervix, 35, 37
change, 103
chest, 30
Circles at the Doorstop technique,
  80
circulation issues, 134
cleanliness, 65, 87, 111
clitoral head, 33
clitoral hood, 32, 34
clitoral legs, 33
clitoral/non-penetrative
  techniques, 71–79
clitoral shaft, 33
clitoridectomies, 11
clitoris, 22, 31, 33, 34, 130, 143
clothing, 50
coconut oil, 67
compliments, 50
confidence, 17, 21, 44
connections, 50
contrasts, 94
control, 140–141

cul-de-sac, 35
cultural messages, 54, 56

D

dancing, 51, 138
deep breaths, 57, 120, 137
dementia, 21
Digging for Pleasure technique, 84
dildos, 107, 108
disabilities, 47–48
distractions, 57, 132, 133, 139, 142
Diva Wash, 111
Dodson, Betty, 56
Double-Dipping Technique, 84
double standards, 27
Double Up technique, 83
douching, 38
dressing up, 50
drugs, 134

E

earlobes, 30
eating, 50, 51–52
elastomer, 97
electric toothbrush, 92
emotional issues, 52–53
endorphins, 19, 127
erogenous zones
  defined, 29
  exploration of, 27–35, 143
  genitals, 31–35
  non-genital, 29–31
erotic books, 51
erotic games, 160–165
erotic potential, enhancing your,
  44–61
estrogen, 40, 58
exercise, 51, 138
exercise-induced orgasms (EIOs), 87
Exhibitionist and Voyeur game, 162
expectations, 52
experimentation, 65, 111, 143

F

fake orgasms, 155
fantasies, 115–117, 157

feathers, 93
feet, 31
female anatomy, 31–35
female ejaculation, 82, 83, 146
female sexuality, 54, 56
feminist movement, 56
Feminist Porn Awards, 60
fertility, 47
Fifty Shades of "Do As I Say" game,
  164
Figure Eight technique, 75
films, 118
Finger Play technique, 86
fingers, 31
flirting, 50
food, 51–52
foreskin, 34
Form 2 vibrator, 106
full-body toys, 93

G

gay men, 18
genitals, 31–35
Glide and Twist technique, 78
glycerin, 68
Going in Circles technique, 79
Got Your Clit technique, 77
G-spot
  existence of, 24, 144
  finding, 36
  location of, 32, 35
  orgasms, 81, 83, 84, 145–149
G-spot and Clitoris technique, 83
guilt, 10, 140

H

hands, 31
head, 30
health benefits, 14, 19, 21, 55
Her-Job technique, 76
Hitachi Magic Wand, 98
hormones, 58, 66, 133
human papilloma virus (HPV), 19, 48
hypogastric nerve, 128

I

imagination, 115
immune system, 21
impatience, 139
Ina 2 vibrator, 103
infections, 38
infertility, 47
inner arm, 30
inner lips, 32
inner thighs, 31
insecurities, 45
insomnia, 19, 21
intersex, 34

J

Jacuzzi jets, 91
journaling, 59, 138
Justisse Method, 37

L

labia, 32, 34
Labia Roll technique, 72
Lap Dance, 163
latex toys, 97
Leaf Vitality, 105
legs, relaxing your, 122
lesbian women, 18
libido
    arousal and, 58–59
    boosting your, 49–53
    changes in, 58
    factors affecting, 58
lifestyle habits, 53
lingerie, 50
Liv 2 vibrator, 100
location, 116
Long-Distance Love, 161
lubricants, 19, 20, 41
    choosing, 67
    ingredients in, 68
    need for, 65, 66, 140
    oil-based, 67
    silicone-based, 67
    water-based, 67
Luna Beads, 109, 121

M

makeup brushes, 93
mantras, 56, 137, 140
Mardi Gras beads, 93
Mardi Gras Rabbit, 107
massagers, 92, 93
masturbation. *See also* self-
    pleasure
    benefits of, 14–21, 55
    compared with partner sex, 17, 26
    in different locations, 116
    easing into, 54–61
    feelings about, 131, 134
    finding time for, 20
    history of, 10–11
    importance of regular, 61
    mixed messages about, 54, 56
    with partner, 160–165
    positions for, 69, 116
    promotion of, 11
    statistics on frequency of, 9, 55,
        149
    stigma surrounding, 11, 19
    techniques, 70–87
medications, 53, 66, 132
meditation, 137
men
    erogenous zones in, 27–28
    masturbation by, 9, 27–28
menopause, 40–41, 66
Mia 2 vibrator, 106
mind
    as sexual organ, 142
    wandering, 139
mons pubis, 32
mood setting, 118–119
multiple orgasms, 143

N

Naked Mime game, 165
neck, 30
negative messages, 131, 134,
    138–139, 140, 153–154
nerves, 128

New Relationship Energy (NRE), 58
nipple clamps, 109, 122
nonoxynol-9, 111
non-vibrating toys, 108–109
notebooks, 57
nutrition, 51–52

O

oil-based lubricants, 67
opening of vagina, 34
Open the Cupboards technique, 73
Orchid Mood Frisky vibrator, 100
orgasm
    building up to, 123
    emphasis on, 126
    exercise-induced, 87
    experience of, 126, 127, 130
    factors affecting, 132–134
    faking, 155
    giving yourself permission for,
        140–141
    G-spot, 81, 83, 84, 145–149
    lack of, 131–132, 157–158
    learning to, 17
    multiple, 143
    during partner sex, 152–158
    phases of, 129–130
    physical strategies for reaching,
        142–143
    relaxing your legs and, 122
    savoring experience of, 141
    stuck on edge of, 136
    types of, 128
    ways to improve your, 137–143
Original Magic Wand, 98
outer lips, 32, 34
overstimulation, 139
oxytocin, 19, 127, 148

P

pain, 65
painful sex, 53, 78, 79
pain management, 47–48
pain relief, 21
paintbrushes, 93

palms, 31
pampering, 57
parabens, 68, 111
parenthood, 52
partner sex, 17, 18, 26, 152–165
    inability to orgasm and, 155
    incorporating masturbation into,
        152–153
    orgasm during, 152–158
    Q&A, 152–160
    sex toys and, 159–160
    solo sex games and, 160–165
pelvic floor exercises, 121
pelvic floor muscles, 21, 109, 127
pelvic nerve, 128
pelvic rocking, 121
penis, 34
performance anxiety, 154
perineal sponge, 34, 84
Perineal Sponge technique, 80
perineum, 34, 101
Persistent Genital Arousal Disorder
    (PGAD), 128
personal issues, 53
phthalates, 97
physical conditions, 53
physical techniques, 120–123
Planned Parenthood, 11
playfulness, 114–115
pleasure points, 122. *See also*
    erogenous zones
pleasure seeking, 50–51
pornography, 60
positions, 69, 116
positives, 49, 57
positive thinking, 137
post-pregnancy, 40
post-surgery, 48–49
prayer, 137
pregnancy, 38, 133
pressure to perform, 133
privacy, 57
Progressive Pleasure Club, 94
progressive relaxation, 57, 138
prolactin, 127, 148

puberty, 37
public places, 116, 121
pudendal nerve, 128
Pure Wang, 108

Q

Quattro Butt Plug, 107

R

rabbit ears, 102
rape fantasies, 115
relationship issues, 52–53
relaxation, 57, 58, 115, 134, 137–138, 154
religion, 19
repetition, 103
resentment, 133
resources, 168–169
rhythm, 136
Rock and Roll technique, 76

S

scalp, 30
scrotum, 34
self-awareness, 138–139
self-esteem, 20, 21, 44, 133
self-hypnosis, 137
self-image, 45–49
self-knowledge, 27
self-pleasure, 11. *See also* masturbation
  dos and don't of, 65
  easing into, 54–61
  giving yourself permission for, 140–141
  initiating, 58–59
  spicing up, 113–123
  talking to partner about, 152–153
  ways to feel good about, 55
senses, 118–119
sex
  defined, 15
  in different locations, 116
  in menopause, 40–41
  painful, 53, 78, 79
  partner, 17, 18, 26, 152–165
  post-pregnancy, 40
  during pregnancy, 38
  as a skill, 24, 26
sex drive. *See* libido
sex education, 14
sex shops, 94
sexsomnia, 74
sex toys
  choosing, 19–20
  cleaning, 65, 87, 111
  factors to consider in, 96–97
  full-body toys, 93
  household objects as, 91–93
  materials of, 96–97
  need for, 109
  non-vibrating, 108–109
  partner sex and, 159–160
  power of, 96
  sharing of, 19
  for two, 101
  use of, 140
  vibrators, 98–107
  where to buy, 94
sexual attractiveness, 47
sexual intercourse, 15, 24
sexuality, 44, 54, 56
sexually transmitted infections (STIs), 19, 48
sexual organs
  differentiation of, 34
  female, 31–35
sexual pleasure, 15, 140–141
sexual relationships, 15, 17. *See also* partner sex
sexual self, 44
shame, 14, 56
shoulders, 30
Show and Tell game, 164
showerheads, 91
silicone-based lubricants, 67
silicone toys, 97, 108
simultaneous orgasms, 153–154
sleep, 19, 21, 148
smell, 119
soap, 111
solo sex, 11. *See also* masturbation; self-pleasure

sound, 118, 120
Squeeze Tease technique, 75
squirting, 82, 146
stigma, 11, 19
stress, 21, 58, 133, 137
Stroke of Pleasure technique, 71
Stronic Zwei Pulsator, 101
supplements, 52

T

taboos, 117
taste, 119
Tease the Rosebud technique, 85
teasing, 122–123
techniques, 70–87
  anal, 85–87
  clitoral/non-penetrative, 71–79
  physical, 120–123
  vaginal, 80–84
terminology, 11, 26
testicles, 34
testosterone, 58, 134
textiles, 93
textures, 93, 94, 96
Three-Finger Massage, 74
Three Oranges and a Lemon game, 153
Tiger, 105
time, 57, 116, 123, 132, 140
tiredness, 133
to-do lists, 138
toes, 31
touch, 118
Tread Lightly technique, 72
trust, 65

U

urethral opening, 32
urethral sponge, 35
urinary tract infections (UTIs), 21, 67, 87
urination, 141
U-spot, 32

V

vagina, 24, 26, 31, 34–35, 38

vaginal discharge, 37
vaginal dryness, 66
vaginal lubrication, 66
vaginal techniques, 80–84
vaginismus, 79
vagus nerve, 128, 129, 137
Vanity Rabbit, 102
vestibular bulbs, 33, 34, 143
vibrators
  addiction to, 99
  choosing, 110
  vs. dildos, 107
  during menopause, 41
  types of, 98–107
visual ambiance, 118
vulva, 24, 31, 32

W

Waking Up technique, 71
washing machines, 92
water-based lubricants, 67
Wellbutrin, 132
We-Vibe 4 Plus, 104, 121
Windows to the Soul game, 165
Windshield Wiper technique, 75
women
  erogenous zones in, 27–28
  masturbation by, 9, 27–28
women-friendly porn, 60

Y

yeast infections, 38
youth, 47

CPSIA information can be obtained
at www.ICGtesting.com
Printed in the USA
LVHW050323100419
613526LV00004B/4/P

9 781592 336791